THE WOMAN'S GUIDE TO SEX ON THE WEB

Also by Anne Semans and Cathy Winks
The New Good Vibrations Guide to Sex

Edited by Anne Semans and Cathy Winks
Sex Toy Tales

THE WOMAN'S GUIDE TO SEX ON THE WEB

Anne Semans and Cathy Winks

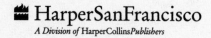
HarperSanFrancisco
A Division of HarperCollinsPublishers

HarperCollins Web Site: http://www.harpercollins.com

HarperCollins®, and HarperSanFrancisco™ are trademarks of HarperCollins Publishers Inc.

HarperCollins books may be purchased for educational, business, or sales promotional use. For information please write: Special Markets Department, HarperCollins Publishers, Inc., 10 East 53rd Street, New York, NY 10022.

FIRST EDITION

Designed by Jessica Shatan

Library of Congress Cataloging-in-Publication Data
Semans, Anne.
   The woman's guide to sex on the Web / Anne Semans and Cathy Winks.
Includes index.
   ISBN 0–06–251548–9 (pbk.)
   1. Computer sex. 2. Women's computer network resources.
   I. Winks, Cathy. II. Title.
   HQ23.W485 1999
   025.06'3067—dc21   98–35066

---

99 00 01 02 03 ❖ RRD (H) 10 9 8 7 6 5 4 3 2 1

To Roxanne, a future surfer

Contents

Acknowledgments

Heartfelt thanks to Jane Duvall for leads, encouragement, advice, and friendship. The online community is a welcoming one, and we're grateful to the following people for information, advice, and referrals. Special thanks to all those who took time out of their busy schedules to grant us phone and e-mail interviews.

Thanks to Marie Acacia, Kim Airs, Anaheed Alani, Isadora Alman, Madeleine Altmann, Anne747, Danni Ashe, Ellen Barnard, Marianna Beck, Todd Belton, Adrienne Benedicks, Indina Beuche, Joani Blank, Brad Borevitz, Gloria Brame, Susie Bright, Cara Bruce, Krissy Cababa, Margaret Campbell, Asia Carrera, Bruce Collen, Al Cooper, Ph.D., Janis Maria Cortese, Geneva Daniel, Brad Davis, Genevieve Field, Angelo Gagliardi, Dr. Sandor Gardos, Kelly Garland, Katharine Gates, Jack Hafferkamp, Steven Kapelow, T. L. Kelly, Debby Levinson, Bobby Lilly, L. Michelle, Mary Anne Mohanraj, Christophe Pettus, Jeff Phillips, Deborah Puckett, Cornelia Read, Gene Rohrer, Candida Royalle, Russell from the Society for Human Sexuality, Judy Siefer, Ph.D., Edie Solow, Annie Sprinkle, Andrew Sullivan, Joan Kennedy Taylor, Laura Tisoncik, Wyyrd, and Katy Zvolerin. And thanks to all the anonymous surfers who filled out our survey—you were our inspiration!

We'd also like to thank Jeff Miller, technical advisor supreme; Michael Castleman for writing advice and encouragement; our agents, Jennie Dunham and Tim Seldes; and our lovely editor, Caroline Pincus.

Anne thanks the Roxanne posse: Sheila, Chris, Cathy, Becky, Trish, Caroline, Jennifer, Genanne, and Jeff; and Cathy thanks Becky most of all.

Introduction

Where can you go to view a turn-of-the-century vibrator, take a peek at porn star Annie Sprinkle's cervix, brush up on sexual technique, or seduce a stranger with words alone? All these unique pleasures and more await you on the World Wide Web.

Thanks to the Web, a user-friendly, multimedia interface that puts the vast resources of the Internet within reach of anyone with access to a computer and modem, millions of women and men around the country are logging on daily in search of information, entertainment, community—and sex, as we're sure you've heard by now. The ready availability of sexually explicit material on the Web has inspired much hand-wringing from the press, politicians, and pundits alike, along with reports that the Internet is filled with lonely guys trolling for nudie photos, that it's virtually dripping with cheesy porn, and that potential addiction and betrayal lurk behind every chat room door. But there's one piece of news that isn't being reported: the Web is actually an unprecedented resource for enhancing women's sex lives.

Not only are women the fastest-growing segment of Web users—up from 16 percent in 1995 to 40 percent in 1998—but over the past decade they've become increasingly influential consumers of all types of adult entertainment. As record numbers of women rent X-rated videos, read erotica, and buy vibrators, the male-dominated adult industry is beginning to respond to their demand for sexually explicit materials that reflect women's experience. But this response has not been fast enough for the female sex activists, performers, entrepreneurs, and consumers who have staked a claim on the virtual frontier—these sexual revolutionaries are using the grassroots, global network of the Web to transform the landscape of erotic expression right here and now.

The accessible, democratic environment of the Web allows women of all ages and backgrounds to create and explore sexually explicit materials that express their authentic desires—they're posting erotic stories, finding resources, and swapping information. In the process, they're discovering a newfound sexual confidence, personal validation, and sense of community that is changing their lives.

Honest Reviews, Provocative Essays

We invite you to join your sister surfers in using the World Wide Web as a forum for sexual expression and a resource for sex-related information. To get you started, we offer opinionated reviews of over two hundred superior sex-related Web sites, chosen for their appeal to women. These sites reflect the broad spectrum of women's sexual desires, while meeting our criteria of originality, accuracy, usefulness, and honesty. Whether your interests lie in erotic entertainment, sex education, parents' resources, community building, or online rendezvous, within these pages you'll find directions to the best sites on the Web.

Through a series of lively essays, interviews, and profiles, we take you on a tour of the steamy side of cyberspace. You'll go behind the scenes with sexperts, adult video stars, and proprietors of women-owned sex toy stores; pick up tips on safe shopping, protecting your privacy, and basic etiquette; and learn how online conferencing and live chat can enrich your sex life and expand your fantasies. But don't take our word for it; let the real experts—the women and men currently enjoying the Web—inspire you with tales of their own erotic adventures. We surveyed approximately two hundred of your fellow surfers; their quotes are included throughout the book and paint a vivid picture of the Web as an exciting and liberating sexual playground.

Your Guide to the Best Sites

Whether you're an experienced surfer or a novice, you may have limited your forays into cybersex because you're either overwhelmed by the sheer volume of sex-related Web sites or turned off by their style and content. The Web is a sprawling, undifferentiated mass of well over a million sites, and surfing can be mind-numbingly tedious if you don't know what to look for or where to look. By far the most visible sex sites online are designed with male consumers in mind, and these commercial sites, with their flashing banner ads promising "live nude girls," are unappealing and often offensive. But for every site offering live video strippers, there's another offering accurate sex information, nonjudgmental advice on sex techniques, cutting-edge erotica, and debates on sexual politics. We'll help you pan for gold in the fast-flowing, ever-expanding stream of information that is the Web, pointing the way to the most useful, titillating, and provocative Web sites created by and for women and couples.

We're motivated to start you on the path to more productive and pleasurable surfing because the rewards of exploring sexual resources on the Web can be so great: increased sexual self-confidence, understanding, and satisfaction. Perhaps you'll discover that sampling new genres of written or visual erotica uncovers desires you never knew you had—or dared to express before. If you've been unsure how to go about that "birds and bees" talk with your child, you can get valuable support and advice from your peers on a parenting site. Your romantic encounters will be even more memorable when you try out toys selected online from a women's sex store or techniques acquired from an online advice column. Before you know it, exposure to the Web's accurate information, sound advice, innovative erotica, and stimulating discussion forums will have raised your comfort level and your sexual IQ tenfold. What's more, you'll probably make quite a few good friends along the way. That's what we mean when we say the Web can change your life.

Who We Are

As you'll soon discover, we're two women with strong opinions, a good sense of humor, and a passionate devotion to freedom of sexual expression. We've spent most of our adult lives writing and talking about sex—as authors of the popular sex manual *The New Good Vibrations Guide to Sex*, editors of the erotic anthology *Sex Toy Tales*, and former vibrator saleswomen at San Francisco's woman-owned erotic emporium Good Vibrations. After over ten years of selling, reviewing, and enjoying sexual materials, we can spot bogus sex information, shoddy sex toys, and formulaic erotica a mile off. By applying our consumer-friendly sensibility to the unparalleled range of sex resources available to women online, we hope to guide you on many satisfying and safe online excursions.

Every self-respecting webmistress includes a rant or two on her site. Rants are about venting your opinion with utter conviction, vehemence, and disregard for objectivity, and they are everywhere in the idiosyncratic, high-decibel environment of the Web. After surfing literally thousands of Web sites, we have some opinions we'd like to put on record ourselves—you'll find them sprinkled throughout the book.

Embrace a World of Pleasure

Over the years, we've fielded thousands of questions about everything from sexual response to spicing up partner sex to selecting lubricants, and we've seen firsthand how access to accurate sex information can enhance anybody's sex life. The Web makes this access possible on a scale previously unimagined, and we're convinced it's a tremendous educational resource that can have a profoundly positive effect on our individual and collective sexual well-being.

You may be concerned that there's something "unnatural" about using the technology of the Web to enhance your sex life, or that expressing interest in any sexual technology is an admission of inadequacy ("I shouldn't *need* that!"). We've encountered variations on this theme throughout our careers as vibrator saleswomen, erotica editors, and cheerleaders for better sex—and our response has always been the same: nothing is more natural than being sexually aroused by mental and physical stimulation—whether this stimulation comes from a vibrator, the sound of your lover's voice, a sensual massage, or an erotic exchange on a computer. When you make arbitrary distinctions between "natural" and "unnatural" sources of stimulation, you simply deny yourself access to that most abundant of natural resources, sexual pleasure.

We see the Web as an amazing sex toy. Like any sex toy, it's a valuable tool for exploring your own sexual preferences, desires, and fantasies. Sure, you don't "need" sexual technology of any kind, any more than you need candlelit dinners, hot baths, four-poster beds, or foot rubs—but don't you deserve it? Imagine how much better the world would be if it were filled with sexually informed and satisfied people—and then go out there and do your bit for a better world. In the inspirational words of sex guru Annie Sprinkle, "Let there be Pleasure on Earth. And let it begin with me!"

Happy Surfing!

ANNE SEMANS

CATHY WINKS

http://www.anneandcathy.com

THE WOMAN'S GUIDE TO SEX ON THE WEB

Chapter One

GETTING STARTED

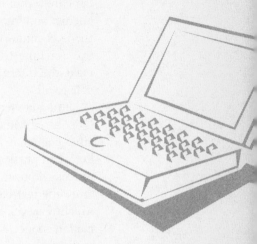

We didn't take shop in high school. And we wrote all our college papers on manual typewriters—back when computers were still exclusively the province of the techno-savvy. Until several years ago, we rarely handled anything more technologically complex than an electric vibrator. So we consider ourselves living proof that you don't need a degree in computer science to enjoy a lusty romp on the Web. All you need is some basic equipment, curiosity, and an adventurous spirit. In this chapter, we'll review the tools and terminology that will help you get started online.

The Internet and the Web

For most of us, the origins of online communication are so hazy that it's almost as though "in the beginning God said, let there be the Internet." Actually a far-from-divine entity, namely, the U.S. Department of Defense, created the Internet in the late 1960s as a military communications tool that could remain operational in the event of a nuclear war. Basically, the Internet connects a vast array of computer networks via phone lines—both its own high-speed pathways and standard phone lines. From the get-go, this system was completely decentralized, so that the lines of communication would be less susceptible to attack from our cold-war "enemies." This same absence of a central authority survives in the anarchic environment of today's Web.

Federal funding subsidized the expansion of the Internet, which grew to link a global community of government agencies, scientists, research institutions, and universities. Throughout the '80s, members of this technical elite benefited from the worldwide contacts, electronic messaging, group conferencing, and information sharing that the Internet allowed. By the late '80s, the U.S. military moved on to high-security networks of its own, paving the way for unrestricted public access to the Internet. The time was ripe to make the Internet's networking, educational, and research possibilities available to all.

Until quite recently, you had to be somewhat of a techno-geek to master the Unix-based syntax required to navigate the Internet. In order to make this powerful communications medium more accessible to the average citizen, a European physics lab developed the technology for the user-friendly, graphical interface known as the World Wide Web. The Web is an overlay that transforms the text-based environment of the Internet into a multimedia display in which text, graphics, audio, and video can be combined into "pages" of information connected by "hyperlinks" that allow surfers to roam from topic to topic at the click of a mouse. Its dazzling multimedia and interactive capabilities, and the fact that it has put the vast resources of the Internet within reach of anyone with access to a personal computer and a modem, have earned the Web the status of being one of the most significant inventions of the twentieth century.

Technically speaking, the Web is a subset of the Internet, but thanks to its versatility and ease of use, it has quickly become the dominant online medium—and it could well be the fastest-growing communications medium of all time. These days, when people refer to the "Internet" or the "Net," chances are good they're actually referring to the Web. As of this writing, there are over fifty million people using the Web, and their numbers are increasing every day. If ever there was a bandwidth—oops, we mean bandwagon—to climb aboard, this is definitely the one. Here's how *you* can get on board.

Hardware and Software

Setting Up
You'll need the following basic hardware and software to access the Web.

Computer
Obviously, a computer is the first thing you need. PC fans should start with no less than a 486 processor (but Pentiums are optimal), and Mac users will need either a 68040 or a Power PC processor. You may be able to get by with eight megabytes of RAM, but be prepared to buy more if you want to

take full advantage of Web features such as streaming video or real-time chat. A color monitor is essential to appreciate Web visuals, and you'll want a monitor that allows you to fit an entire Web page on your screen without having to scroll around to take it all in: a fifteen-inch monitor should do the trick.

Modem

Modems transmit data from one computer to another over phone lines. Most computers these days come with internal modems preinstalled, or you can buy an external modem. Modem speed can make or break your online experience. The faster the modem, the faster it will transfer Web pages onto your computer screen, and the less time you'll spend twiddling your thumbs on the "World Wide Wait." Graphics, photos, and videos take up greater *bandwidth*—the term for the amount of data that can be transmitted through any online channel—than text, and if you want to enjoy any of these features in less time than it takes to grow gray hairs, you owe it to yourself to invest in the fastest modem you can afford. Speeding up access to the Web is the biggest technological challenge facing Internet service providers, and you can rest assured that phone, cable TV, and high-tech companies are all working (and competing) on ways to expand bandwidth and minimize gridlock on overcrowded phone lines.

In the meantime, we all have to make do with the current technology. We researched this book using a 33.6-Kbps modem ("bps" stands for "bits per second"), and you shouldn't settle for less. Just be aware that by the time this book is published, 56-Kbps modems may well be the standard. Currently, you also have the option of using an ISDN modem; these are much faster than standard modems, but they entail higher monthly fees and the expense of installing the digital phone lines they require. A new technology called DSL (Digital Subscriber Technology) promises to use ordinary phone lines to transmit data at a speed over thirty times faster than that of traditional modems, but it's not yet affordable for most consumers.

If you work in a high-tech office or live in an urban area that caters to high-tech workers, you may have access to a T1 line, an Internet pathway that is exponentially faster than standard phone lines. These are too expensive to install in the average home, but some apartment buildings in high-tech centers such as New York or San Francisco are beginning to offer T1 access to entice prospective renters, much as they used to offer cable TV.

If you plan on spending a lot of time online, you should consider adding a second, dedicated phone line for your modem; otherwise, you'll miss a lot of calls from your friends and family. Plus, as we found while researching this book, there's no greater luxury than surfing the Web and chatting on the phone with your co-author at the same time! If you stick with just one phone line, we recommend getting a voice mail system so callers won't get a busy signal. Finally, if you have call waiting, do disable it before going online, or you'll be disconnected from the Web whenever someone calls you.

Communications Software

Simply put, the communications software is the program that instructs your modem to dial up your connection to the Internet. Usually your Internet service provider will supply you with the communications software necessary to get online, or it will be packaged with your modem. Computer stores also sell universal communications software packaged with offers for free trial hours of Internet access.

Internet Service Providers (ISPs)

Most people access the Internet through centralized computer systems known as ISPs. You dial into the ISP, which links you to the Internet via its own high-speed connection. ISPs usually supply you with the browser software you'll need to view the Web and to send e-mail. Since the Web's popularity has spawned an entire industry of ISPs, you won't have any trouble finding one—just look in the Yellow Pages, or check the ads in local papers and computer or business magazines. The quality and service of ISPs can vary greatly, and we encourage you to shop around (see the sidebar "Choosing an Internet Service Provider," p. 5).

Commercial Online Services

An alternative to ISPs, commercial online services such as America Online (AOL), Microsoft Network (MSN), Prodigy, and CompuServe are popular with first-timers because they provide an easy-to-use, well-defined online environment. You dial directly into the service, which has its own proprietary software and content: news, shopping, general information, and members-only chat rooms and discussion groups. While they offer access to the Web, some commercial services reserve the right to filter potentially "offensive" materials, which can be particularly problematic if you're interested in sexual materials.

Web Browser Software

Browser software allows you to explore the Web and transforms the programming language of a Web site into a multimedia experience. You can't admire clever graphics, drool over sexy photos, or follow hyperlinks without it. Browsers feature convenient navigational buttons, organizational tools (so you can save and sort information on your favorite sites), and editing options (useful when you want to cut and paste information from a Web page to another file). Netscape Navigator and Microsoft Internet Explorer

CHOOSING AN INTERNET SERVICE PROVIDER

Here are some things to consider when deciding which ISP to sign up with:

Rates. First, figure out how much time you expect to spend online. Some ISPs offer a flat monthly rate for unlimited use, others charge by the hour, and many will let you choose between the two. Choose the plan that best suits your needs.

Speed. How fast is their connection to the Internet? Your ISP should use at least a T1 line, and you can rejoice if they've got a T3 (which is even faster). After all, your own spiffy fast modem will slow to a crawl if you dial into an ISP with an Internet connection that's slower than yours!

Location. Make sure your ISP is local. The beauty of the Internet is that you can communicate with anyone in the world for the price of a local phone call. Don't blow that by signing up with an ISP that's outside your area code. Most ISPs and commercial online services offer local access numbers, but if you live in a remote area you should double-check before signing up. If you plan on accessing the Internet a lot while traveling, you should look for an ISP that offers an 800 number or has local numbers virtually everywhere.

Privacy. Ask about their policy on privacy and confidentiality. It's standard practice for ISPs not to make your name and address accessible to the public, but it's best to double-check.

Service. Find out how long the ISP has been in business, and ask for references. Since there is so much competition for your business, many will give you a free trial period. Try their service during peak hours (all day on weekends, and weekdays after 5:00 p.m.), to make sure you can get online. Before you sign up, call or e-mail with a few questions just to get a feel for their customer service. You can ask what their technical support hours are, how best to contact the company, whether browser and communications software are included when you sign up, and how user-friendly their installation instructions are.

Referrals. What do your friends like? Nothing beats a glowing referral from a friend. Co-workers and computer business owners are also good sources for recommendations.

are the most commonly used browsers; you can download these (as well as any new releases) for free off Netscape and Microsoft's own Web sites.

Miscellaneous Plug-Ins

Once you're actually exploring the Web, you'll periodically encounter some feature—maybe it's an audio clip, a bit of video, or a compressed document—that won't function unless you install an enabling program, called a *plug-in*. Many sites will link you to instructions on downloading and installing these free plug-ins.

Other Ways to Get Online

If setting up your own Internet access sounds too expensive or time-consuming, you do have other options. Cafés and copy shops in many cities offer Internet access for an hourly fee, and renting time on the Web can be a great way to test the waters. Libraries are now outfitted with computer terminals that have Internet access, but these terminals may take you to text-only versions of Web sites. Of course, if you're on a quest for sex-related sites, you might prefer a little more privacy than these options afford! Many universities offer free Internet accounts to students and faculty, a perk you should definitely avail yourself of if you qualify. Couch potatoes might want to look into buying a WebTV, which allows you to surf the Web through your TV, using a remote control. As yet, WebTVs have more limited capabilities than computers; for instance, you won't have access to most Web-based chat rooms.

Vernacular

The following crash course in Web vocabulary will make a whole lot more sense once you actually go online. With a little exposure, these terms will become second nature to you—you'll soon be "bookmarking URLs" at every turn. Like any new technology, the Web has its own jargon. For a quick definition of any of the Web-specific terms you'll find throughout this book, check out the Glossary.

Your destination on the World Wide Web is known as a *Web site*. Most sites are made up of separate *Web pages*, and the entry page or table of contents page for each Web site is referred to as its *homepage*.

Hypertext links are the most uniquely defining feature of the Web. These allow you to travel within a page, within a site, or from one site to another at the click of a mouse. The hyperlink, usually referred to simply as a *link*, can be embedded in an icon, a word, a phrase, or an image that is highlighted in some way (appearing in a different color, in bold, or underlined); when you click on the link, it catapults you to your next destination. For example, say you're at a sex site reading an article about masturbation. The author may provide links within the article that transport you to other pages of that same site where you can read famous quotes about masturbation or a list of books on the subject, and she may also provide links that send you to an entirely different site where you can shop for sex toys. You can choose to stay on the original page or to follow the links and see where they lead you. The word *Web* really is an apt metaphor for this nonlinear network of linked pages.

It's not uncommon to get so caught up in following a trail of interesting links that you get distracted from your original goal and wind up wandering all over the map. Fortunately, your browser comes with a couple of handy features that will help you and Toto find your way back to Kansas. You can tag any page you like with a *bookmark*, which will store that page's address in a folder so you can return to it later. This bookmark will remain in the folder even after you turn off your computer. During a single surfing session, your browser will also create a documented history of the pages you've visited, so you can return to any one in the string by clicking on its address.

Every Web page possesses a unique address, known as its *URL* (uniform resource locator). When you type any given URL into the address window of your browser, off you'll go to that page. Even if you've never been on the Web, you've probably seen URLs on everything from advertisements to business cards to book jackets; they're distinguished by a string of words, letters, and punctuation marks that looks like this: http://www.anneandcathy.com. For all you nerd wannabes, here's a basic dissection of a typical URL address:

The "http://" stands for *hypertext transfer protocol* and indicates that you're dealing with a Web address (versus a gopher, newsgroup, or FTP). "Protocol" refers to the language used to transmit files over the Internet, and in this instance hypertext files are being transferred.

The "www." refers to a Web site's host computer, also known as its server. While not every Web address includes "www," which stands for "World Wide Web," it is a common convention.

"Anneandcathy.com" is the *domain name*, the identifying name chosen and registered by the individual, company, organization, or two nice girls who created the page. The first part of the domain name is referred to as the *unique domain*, and the suffix (in this case ".com") is the *top-level domain*.

Top-level domains provide a way of sorting the vast array of Web sites into general categories. Currently, only a handful of these suffixes are commonly used: "com," or commercial, "org," organizational, "edu," educational, and "net" for networks such as ISPs. By far the most common one you'll encounter when surfing for sex-related sites is "com." An expanded list of top-level domain names is currently in the works to fulfill the need for a more detailed classification system.

You'll notice that many of the URLs listed in this book are lengthy and loaded with backslashes. The slashes indicate different subsections of a Web site; for instance, http://www.anneandcathy.com is our site's homepage, but http://www.anneandcathy.com/petpeeves could be a page full of Anne's petty annoyances and http://www.anneandcathy.com/petpeeves/pets could be a page specifically devoted to her peeve about the number of sites that post photos of their creators' cats. If you try surfing to a Web page with a long address and get the message "file not found," you can try entering the shortest version of the URL up through the top-level domain to check whether the site itself is gone or whether that particular page has simply been taken down (perhaps Anne has had a change of heart after finally experiencing a cat's true affection and has taken down her "pet peeve about pets" page).

Web addresses change with the wind, so don't be surprised if several of the URLs in this book lead you to a dead end. Fortunately, some handy resources remedy this situation. If you're looking for the address of a particular site, you can use a *search engine*, which searches the Web for matches to whatever name or phrase you specify. If you're looking for information on a general topic and don't have a specific site in mind, you can use a *directory*, which organizes site listings into general categories. We'll expand more on these two powerful research tools in chapter 8, "Directories, Search Engines, and Links," where you'll also find pointers for refining your search.

Assistance

We could fill up an entire page just cataloging the various technical mishaps we experienced while writing this book: in one month alone, Cathy's computer froze up every time she tried to enter a chat room, Anne's phone lines went dead during heavy rains, and we both suffered the fate of our ISPs going down for a couple of days at a stretch. If you know where to go for help, you can save yourself quite a bit of time and frustration.

• Your ISP offers technical support and should provide trained phone staffers who can walk you through any problems related to your account (without making you feel like an idiot!). Select your ISP based on the quality and availability of their customer service—even if their rates are a little higher. It's worth it to be able to contact a human being when you need assistance.

• Manuals are a logical place to look if you're having problems with your hardware or software. If you can't find an answer to your question in the manual, try the company's technical support number, or, if you still have access, visit their Web site.

• Ask your friends for referrals if you're thinking about investing in computer equipment or signing up with an ISP. Test drive their setup to see if it meets your needs.

• Computer store staff can answer your questions about hardware, software, and getting online, as well as provide you with tips on establishing a local Internet account.

• Seek assistance from the source. If you've got browser questions or want to download recent upgrades, go to the company's Web site:
Netscape http://www.netscape.com
Microsoft Internet Explorer http://www.microsoft.com

Now that you've got the fundamentals under control, you're ready to go out and give Web surfing a whirl. Allow us to congratulate you on taking a communications tool invented by the U.S. military and using it for sexual entertainment. If that's not national pride, we don't know what is!

Chapter Two

Arts and Entertainment

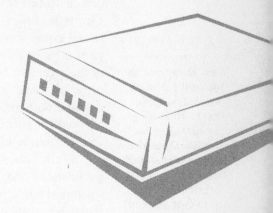

Once upon a Time

Until quite recently, erotic literature presumed a male readership, and erotic art catered to a male gaze. For all most pornographic writers and filmmakers seemed to care, women seeking realistic depictions of female pleasure could go look in a mirror. Any woman who wanted to curl up with a sexy periodical had to settle for mainstream men's magazines filled with nudie pix and entertaining but far-fetched letters to the editor. Tame spin-offs "for the ladies," such as *Playgirl*, somehow managed to miss the boat. But then, something wonderful happened.

Everybody's heard of the sexual revolution of the '60s, but few stop to consider the revolution in sexual expression that took place twenty years later when desktop publishing and video technology burst onto the scene. These relatively low-cost, accessible technologies democratized the production of written and visual erotica. Suddenly, anyone with imagination and vision could put together a periodical or shoot a video. Sexual perspectives seldom represented before—those of women, gays and lesbians, S/M mavens, and others—found their way onto paper and videotape and eventually into homes all across the country. While democracy has a downside (we all have an equal right to create erotica, but not all erotica is created equally well), the explosion of new voices and new visions brought an unprecedented range and diversity of sexual representations into the mainstream.

These technological developments coincided with an era of intense debate within the women's community about sexually explicit materials. During the so-called feminist porn wars, those who embraced freedom of sexual expression faced off against those who subscribed to the view that all porn is inherently degrading to women. As a result, women on either side of the argument began struggling to define their own relationship to sexual materials, to actively explore their own sexual desires and fantasies, and to describe authentic female experience. An increasing number of women adopted the attitude that if you don't like the sexually explicit materials you see, you should go out and make some of your own.

And they did—the late '80s became a heyday for both alternative adult publications and women-written erotica. While book publishers initially stuck to the relative gentility of works such as *Ladies Own Erotica* or Lonnie Barbach's women-authored anthologies, alternative magazine publishers had the flexibility and the audacity to experiment with a wide range of subject matters and styles.

Suddenly, women in search of a simple erotic thrill no longer had to slog through images of airbrushed perfection, articles about stereo components, or goofy cartoons. Whether you were drawn to the sophistication of *Libido* magazine's "literary erotica for eggheads," the irreverent exuberance of *On Our Back*'s "entertainment for the adventurous lesbian," the elegant aesthetics of *Yellow Silk*, or the transgressive fiction of *Frighten the Horses*, chances were very good you'd find a magazine suited to your tastes. From erotic poetry to down-and-dirty raunch, female authors delivered the goods to an appreciative audience of women and men.

Alas, very few of the innovative erotic magazines of the '80s survived the high costs of print publication, the difficulties of nailing down reliable printers, and the perils of attempting to distribute adult materials beyond the adult bookstore circuit. Today, alternative periodicals struggle to muster both the circulation and the advertisers required to stay afloat. Despite a sea change in societal attitudes, reflecting a growing acceptance of sexual media by ordinary men and women, the country's legal climate—from the chilling effects of the Meese Commission to the confusing implications of the latest Child Protection Acts—isn't hospitable to mom-and-pop erotica publishers.

Despite the difficulties of the marketplace, one simple fact remains: the genie of innovative sexual expression can't be stuffed back into a bottle. Women's erotic voices can't be restricted to book-of-the-month club prose,

"I am always on the lookout for some candid, graphic, heart-thumping sexual sites for couples. Ones that involve pictures of beautiful men and women, but real ones—not sixteen-year-old Barbies and fifty-year-old males."

and cutting-edge erotica hasn't disappeared; it's simply morphed into online form, expanding the boundaries of sexual entertainment on the World Wide Web. In this chapter, we explore how an erotic aesthetic that includes and celebrates women's voices is thriving in cyberspace.

Some Like It Hot: Online Erotica

Imagine a group of strangers sitting in your living room having this conversation:

"The character development in this story was great, and I nearly came myself during the vivid description of Nancy's face during orgasm, but I just didn't buy the explosive orgasm she had while doing jumping jacks," says one person.

"Yeah, I agree. I didn't find that sex scene very believable—it might have worked if we knew Nancy was easily orgasmic or had *ben wa* balls inside her," says another.

"Oh come on, who orgasms from *ben wa* balls?" asks yet another. "No, no, the scene would be more realistic if Nancy came from lying on top of her vibrator."

Sound like an unlikely scenario? It is. Sure, these days you can join a reading group organized by friends, the library, or even Oprah Winfrey, but don't expect to find any erotica on the recommended reading list. After all, sex is something we do behind closed doors and haven't learned to talk about in public. Most of us find it hard enough to articulate our sexual desires and share them with a partner, let alone total strangers. Besides, if you are brave enough to confess your preference for leather-clad female protagonists at your neighborhood reading group, you might wind up on the receiving end of some pretty hostile (or lewd) stares during your next trip to the grocery store.

Now imagine that the conversation just described is taking place in a virtual living room. You communicate with dozens of other participants about your favorite erotic tale by simply tapping away at your keyboard. You can't see the others, nor can they see you. You might not even know their gender. No one knows who you are, so you feel free to describe exactly what turns you on.

Welcome to online erotica forums—gatherings of men and women who like to exchange thoughts electronically about all kinds of erotica. Sometimes the discussions are posted to a specific Web site, and sometimes they take place among e-mail subscribers to a free mailing list (called a *list-serv*). Erotica forums aren't necessarily limited to discussions of fiction. In the Erotica Readers Association (ERA), participants can swap lyrics from sexy songs, rate scenes from R- and X-rated films, or just discuss whatever sparks their libido. The commercial online service CompuServe offers forums on erotic poetry and romance novels. Some erotica forums also host writing workshops.

Why Women Are Getting Hooked

Erotica forums appeal to women for several reasons. Foremost is anonymity. In 1996, Adrienne Benedicks and Donna Newman-Ayala founded the ERA, a forum and listserv that focuses on erotica with a "woman's view of sensuality." Since then, the group's membership has climbed to over one hundred members, most of whom are women. Adrienne explains, "Once women realized they wouldn't be recognized, that people weren't going to say 'ooh, look at her—she writes erotica, she's such a slut,' they started signing up."

Forums provide a safe place for women to write about or discuss sex openly, which can have unexpected benefits. "Forums are a wonderful way for women to explore their sexuality. Expressing yourself to other women in

---

A WORD ABOUT COPYRIGHT

Any material published on the Web is essentially broadcast around the world, and the unfortunate downside of this wide exposure is the potential for copyright infringement. If your erotic writing or photography appears online, it's a safe bet that at some point you'll run across your work posted on another site without attribution. Not all copyright violations are intentional: sometimes material is simply passed from friend to friend and ends up on another site without a credit attached. Usually your request to remove or credit the piece will be honored, but many adult pay site owners routinely post stolen work, exploiting the fact that most artists don't bother prosecuting copyright cases because they are costly, time-consuming and not—to date—financially rewarding.

Unfortunately, many online authors respond to this state of affairs by restricting what they're willing to publish for public consumption. As Geneva Daniel of *screech* comments, "I think the reason there are so few sites with decent content out there is because of the high incidence of intellectual theft—it prevents me from posting some of my favorite work, as these stories are near and dear to me and it would pain me to see them collected at some random, screaming, blinking sex site."

However, as the Web becomes a more mainstream—and therefore more legislated—communications medium, the technology that enables artists to track online violations of copyright will become cheaper and more widely used. It's already possible to digitally encrypt copyright and permission information, and some photographers tag their work with digital watermarks. These precautions are obviously of particular interest to artists, who are accustomed to being paid for reprint rights.

If you're simply concerned about having control over where your erotica appears, take a common-sense approach and label your work; as Anne of Anne's Erotic Story Archives points out, "Don't give anyone the excuse to say, 'I didn't know you would object.'" Once Anne adopted the following tactics, the rate at which her stories appeared on pay sites dropped dramatically. "Even with the problems I've encountered, I'm

a faceless communication is great practice for learning to talk to a sexual partner face-to-face," says Adrienne. Women are reveling in this newfound freedom, as evidenced by this participant: "We fantasize as much as men, but society teaches us that 'good girls don't, bad girls do.' Now, with the opening of the erotica markets, we're just beginning to feel and release our own 'bad girls,' and writing and reading is one way to let go."

The creator of a mailing list known as "Xena's Campfire Girls" rhapsodizes about the liberating aspects of a genre known as "slash fan fiction," in which writers often put a homoerotic or sadomasochistic spin on stories about TV characters. "Slash is basically homegrown, grassroots erotica by and for women," she explains. "Writing slash is an inherently political act—to appropriate the characters of a show and take them places the producers 'won't or can't' go is a self-assertion tool for women, queers, kinky people, and all the disenfranchised het and/or vanilla people unsatisfied by the gender roles and erotic possibilities in mainstream entertainment." For

glad I post my work online," she says. "It's been a wonderful growth experience. I doubt I would be writing at all if it weren't for the Net." Here are a few of Anne's tips for protecting copyright:

• Accompany your piece with a copyright notice, date, your name, and your instructions, such as: "Copyright 1999, Cathy Winks, cathy@anne-andcathy.com. No reposting without express permission of the author." (Bear in mind that including your e-mail address will mean you're more likely to receive unsolicited fan mail as well as permission requests.) You can copyright material published under a pen name.

• Authors should place the copyright notice between the title and the body of the work, and again at the bottom of the work. Anyone copying your work to use on another site will probably cut and paste blocks of text, and they're less likely to cut out the title than a notice at the end of the piece. If you have your own Web site devoted to your work, you may want to copyright the entire site.

• If you write erotica purely for pleasure, you may not care whether it's copied. If you do care,

be selective about where you post online. Avoid Usenet newsgroups, since text and images found in newsgroups are widely—and often correctly—considered to be in the public domain; many pay sites consist entirely of material culled from Usenet postings. You may want to post to smaller groups or private mailing lists (like ERA) that are less visible to the public, or to share your work only with other writers in online workshops. Similarly, you might want to limit your contributions to Web sites that post only copyrighted material.

• Give credit where credit is due! If you want to reprint someone else's work, get their permission first.

• Educate yourself. For a more extensive discussion of these issues, check out these sites:

Ten Big Myths About Copyright Explained
http://www.templetons.com/brad//copymyths.html

U.S. Copyright Office, Library of Congress
http://lcweb.loc.gov/copyright

those interested in reading, writing, or conversing about slash or other erotic fan fiction, Yahoo! has an extensive listing of fan fiction topics.

Of course, many people end up in forums on a quest for new erotic reading material. Sites often post original writing by their contributors, so visitors can sample a variety of styles. Since most forum administrators will post all submissions, the quality of the writing you find may vary wildly. This is one of the only drawbacks of online erotica: you can easily spend hours scrolling through poorly written material, an exercise certain to dampen your desire rather than ignite it. "Some of the stuff in our library is not very good," says Margaret Campbell, a founder of CompuServe's erotica forum. "Some people say the Web is great because it's an even playing field, and there are no editors, but in my experience, editors have a place!"

There are ways to hone in on material that suits your tastes. Since erotica forums are fairly interactive, your best bet is to ask other members for recommendations, or to use the site's list of links as a jumping-off point. If you find authors you like, search for their names to locate more of their material. They might also link to their own favorite writers' work. Generally, you'll find the best writing in online writing workshops, but be prepared to participate!

Style and Content

Some folks wander into an erotica forum or workshop curious about whether there is such a thing as a gender-specific style of writing—a "women's erotica." Erotica readers themselves differ on the answer. While many believe that good writing defies gender, others maintain that there are distinct differences between men's and women's prose. A number of our survey respondents attempted to identify these distinctions. "Women get into feelings while men prefer the visual. Men tend not to spread a scene out over time, but have a need to get to the 'point' more quickly—rather like they do in bed," said one woman. And this man concurs: "Men are more likely to concentrate on the purely physical, women on the physio-emotional." Adrienne Benedicks agrees: "With women writers, it's not just who's fucking whom, it's how and where they're doing it." She believes that one of the benefits of having a coed forum is that the two styles are merging and overall "erotica is becoming much more well-rounded."

As for what people write about—the subject matter runs the gamut. Stories ranging from the romantic to the kinky portray characters of all kinds of sexual persuasions. Workshop writing exercises can be seasonal, yielding a batch of ghoulish stories around Halloween or naughty toy tales at Christmas. If your tastes tend toward a certain theme, whether science fiction smut or gay boys in bondage, you can seek sites devoted to that particular subject.

"I want a good, well-written story. It has to be more than just bodies bumping off each other for me. I like the stories I read to have feeling and a purpose. The characters created on the page should be people, not cardboard cutouts."

Surprisingly enough, there appears to be more self-censorship among participants in online erotica forums and writing workshops than in the print media. Anaïs Nin might have had a tough time cracking this crowd. Many people cite the "big four"—incest, pedophilia, rape, and bestiality—as subjects that should be banned online. When stories on these themes do arise, their fate often lies in the hands of the forum administrator, the webmistress, or a corporate policy. CompuServe's guidelines specifically prohibit any writing on these subjects. The writing workshops offered by Mary Anne Mohanraj (a popular online erotica author) and ERA require potentially offensive material to be flagged, which gives readers the option to pass if they're not interested. According to Adrienne Benedicks, "In ERA, no subject matter is off limits. There are taboo subjects, but I would rather see them coming up and being discussed." The net effect of this informal peer pressure seems to be that even those erotica forums that welcome discussions of potentially troublesome content are more cautious in the long run than many of the individual authors' sites and e-zines reviewed later in this chapter, which tackle some of the most button-pushing topics of the day.

Writing Workshops

Women hoping to hone their smut-writing skills can find encouragement and constructive criticism in online writing workshops. Margaret Campbell says, "Since explicitness is not permitted in CompuServe's 'Hot Romance' forum, our 'Erotica Forum' attracts women hoping to craft the scene that comes after the torrid kiss and passionate embrace." The leap from romance writing to erotica is a short one, since, to satisfy readers, both genres rely on well-crafted seduction and the powerful release of consummation scenes, be they explicit or euphemistic. On her Pink Kink Catalog site, Canadian journalist Donna Laframboise examines several scenes from romance novels as examples of "textual pornography."

Erotic writing workshops flourish online because they provide an easy and convenient way for people to come together, qualities that can be particularly enticing to newcomers. "To find people of a like mind or interest in real life you'd have to ask around, probably embarrassing yourself half to death in the process," explains one workshop participant. "With an online group you enter the space knowing everyone has come with the same intent and they'll let you lurk about timidly in the shadows until you feel like grabbing a chair nearer the front."

Both women and men appreciate the attentiveness and professionalism of participants in the writing workshops offered by sites such as CompuServe and Mary Anne Mohanraj's. Whereas traditional writers' groups may meet once a month with a limited number of people, online workshops offer immediate feedback from dozens of people. For serious writers, this is invaluable. As one ERA member explained, "If I send a piece to be critiqued, I can get feedback within two days. This is important for a writer when the next scene could depend on the response to the first one."

What's more, Adrienne Benedicks claims that because the participants don't discuss their work face-to-face, the criticisms are often more honest: "If you don't have to look at the reaction on someone's face, you're more apt to express your feelings and opinions." Most workshops and forums are governed by rules of etiquette that keep flaming (responding to someone's posted comments with a posting that attacks, insults, or provokes) and inappropriate criticisms to a minimum. Some writing groups are open to readers and writers alike, which appeals to this writer: "The group is not just writers, it's readers—the potential reading public. Gut reaction response can be as valuable as or even more valuable than a formal critique."

Since your real identity need never be revealed, online workshops provide an ideal opportunity for contributors to disguise or change their gender. Some relish the freedom of gender ambiguity. "I use pen names that are gender neutral, not because I'm ashamed or embarrassed about being a woman, but because I think it's more fun for the reader," says one sixty-three-year-old participant. "And it gives me a chance to write from the different perspectives of my various characters. Readers don't know who is talking and therefore have no preconceived idea about what to expect." Others, like this man, enjoy exploiting preconceived notions of gender: "When I write from the female point of view, I find that my story is more accepted if I have a female pen name."

Workshop participants give one another feedback on everything from grammar and plot to whether a story turned them on. "I look for deep characterization, interesting and effective style, a solid plot line, and hot, arousing scenes," says Mary Anne Mohanraj. "Writing that is merely elegant does not make for good erotica. As a tragedy is expected to move the audience to tears, so should erotica be expected to move the audience to arousal."

If you're ready to be moved to arousal, want to learn how to move others to arousal, or just want to talk about arousal, you won't find a more welcoming place than the virtual living rooms known as erotica forums.

Beyond Centerfolds

For sheer mind candy, there's nothing quite as satisfying as a magazine, and erotic magazines can be the most satisfying ones of all. A good erotic magazine delivers a porno buffet: smutty stories, imaginative visuals, provocative commentary, reviews, and advertisements for products and services you won't find in the daily paper. The buffet analogy is especially apt since magazines can offer a tantalizing taste of erotic activities, stimulating appetites you didn't know you had. And the Web affords total, and often totally free, access to a stunning array of magazines. By the way, in this book we'll refer interchangeably to online magazines and e-zines, since it's arbitrary how editors choose to refer to their Web publications.

Toto, We're Not at the Corner Newsstand Any More

Online magazines contain much of the same content as print magazines . . . and then some. Sure, you can find articles, fiction, pictorials, editorials, reviews, and ads, just as in print magazines. But you'll also discover entire community networks, which spiral out in seemingly infinite directions from a single magazine's homepage. You'll be introduced to a diverse cast of characters—flamboyant, pedantic, witty, earnest, outrageous—all of whom have something to say about sex. And you'll be presented with the embarrassment of riches that is every site's list of links. Whether you're seeking more information about S/M, referrals to reputable shopping sites, or recommended erotica sites, every magazine's links page reflects an editorial point of view that can launch you on a uniquely interesting journey.

Online magazines not only provide access to more information, community resources, and thoughtful commentary than you're likely to find at your local newsstand; they also offer a range of taboo-busting erotica that's almost unprecedented offline. In the wake of the Communications Decency Act's defeat, the Web remains one of the least restricted forums for sexual communication this country has ever known. (The CDA was a portion of the Congressional Telecommunications Act of 1996 that would have outlawed all "indecent" materials on the Internet. It was struck down by the Supreme Court in June 1997.) Online publishers don't have to worry about whether printers, distributors, and bookstores will reject their books and magazines based on content, and as a result, they can provide a forum for authors and artists who are exploring transgressive subject matter or who are tired of following the formulaic restrictions of mainstream print publishers. The Web, which knows no boundaries, is proving to be the ideal medium for sexual expression that crosses all boundaries.

Online sex magazines fall into several distinct categories. Some publishers are investing in full-fledged e-zines, modeled on print magazines, with the goal of cultivating brand-name loyalty and carving out a profitable presence on the medium that's predicted to be the dominant communications force of the next century. Others are taking advantage of the Web's unique suitability as a community clearinghouse for members of sexual minorities. Still others are creative individuals thrilled by the opportunity to share their erotic prose with an enormous audience, revel-

Forget masturbation—we've discovered a few design disasters guaranteed to make you go blind.

Reverse Type. Sure, Web sites are a magical blend of text, graphics, audio, and video, but many sites rely first and foremost on the written word. Yet the words themselves get lost in the shuffle astonishingly often, usually due to the mysterious convention of reverse type. You've seen the pages we're talking about—you've probably even tried to read a paragraph or two of vibrant yellow typeface pulsating on a black background before giving up for fear that your overloaded neurons might be shocked into some kind of seizure. Reverse type is pretty and eye-catching. It's great for headers or short quotes. We just would like it to be outlawed whenever more than one hundred consecutive words are involved.

Teeny, Tiny Frames. Here's another example of how site designers sometimes seem to be entertaining themselves in a happy vacuum, blissfully free of concerns such as whether the page is legible. Frame syndrome occurs when a page is divided up into a jigsaw puzzle of geometric sections: a header here, a sidebar there, a banner ad along the bottom, and a table of contents taking up one-third of the screen, each frame complete with its own scroll bars. We've visited sites where, if you wanted to read an erotic story or view a photo, you had to scroll down a frame that took up a mere tenth of the screen. We don't care how big your monitor is—the content should be front and center!

Color Me Sexy. It takes only a few hours of surfing sex sites before a strange sensation overtakes you: Could it be that you're traveling through a color-coded universe? Yes, the code separating "naughty" from "nice" sites is just as strict as the dress code separating biker chicks from Catholic schoolgirls. X-rated sites practically gyrate on your screen with the intensity of their black, red, and yellow color schemes. Educational sites adopt a gentle palette of soothing desert tones—aqua, cream, peach—reminiscent of the Southwestern decor so popular in therapists' offices. And what's the color of choice for those well-intentioned businesses, such as women-owned sex stores, that straddle the line between information and commerce? Lavender does it every time.

ing in what one webmaster refers to as "the international soapbox possibilities" of the Web. Despite their differences, they do all have one thing in common: they relish the experience—and experiment—of sex publishing in cyberspace.

From Zine to Computer Screen

The Web is a haven for hip, antiestablishment periodicals of every variety. In a media world dominated by corporate behemoths, few folks have the resources to get a print magazine off the ground. Sure, if you're JFK, Jr., you have a fighting chance, but where does that leave the rest of us? Many enterprising women and men have responded to the homogeneity of mainstream media by putting together their own paper zines: low-budget, low-production-value broadsheets that reflect the idiosyncrasies of individual editors. They're not in it for the money; they simply want to provide a genuine alternative to the glossies.

Zines of all varieties are flocking online, lured by the Web's relatively low production costs and potentially high exposure. When sexual content is involved, moving online makes all the more sense. As the editors of *mouth organ*—an online zine devoted to sex, gender, and culture—put it: "If we were in print, we'd be a paper zine run off on a photocopier with a *very* limited distribution. Online, in the current atmosphere, we may actually stand a chance of reaching more people, and we don't have to worry about distributors refusing us because of content or about soliciting advertising to stay alive."

Equally appealing to zine publishers and readers is the Web's archiving capability. Periodicals such as the now-defunct *Brat Attack* ("the zine for leatherdykes and other bad girls") don't exactly fit into the Dewey Decimal system and aren't likely to show up in your local library's reading room. Yet, thanks to the miracle of electronic publishing, excellent zines like this one are only a mouse-click away from anyone who visits S/M resource listings online. And many still-existing zines maintain online archives of past issues, providing fans with instant gratification and hours of pleasure.

As is true of paper zines, online magazines sometimes revolve around a single opinionated individual or group of friends who decide, in time-honored Judy Garland–Mickey Rooney fashion, to put on a show! Some of our favorite sites consist of little more than a couple of smart people sounding off with their virtual megaphone. As writer Mary Anne Mohanraj points out, "Online I can find intelligent, open-minded commentary on sexuality that is hard to find in the mainstream world." These authors and editors use their magazines as forums for self-expression, networking, and conducting informal "salons" online. *Mouth organ* editors Todd Belton and Debby Levinson launched their site because "Todd noticed some interesting psychology going on in online environments, had some theories, and realized that you could speculate about this stuff forever. So he started speculating. No one else was doing that kind of material online on a regular basis."

Just as *mouth organ* welcomes comments, critiques, and conversation from readers via its message board, many editors of these salon-style zines find creative ways to interact with their readers. Geneva Daniel of *screech* prints one true-life story submitted by a reader in every issue; Wyyrd of *Hoot Island Graphics* solicits anecdotes about funny things that have happened during sex; and *Venus or Vixen?* features an ongoing erotic story in which the plot twists are guided by readers' e-mail suggestions.

As with all sex sites, a huge number of online magazines are commercial pay sites geared toward men, in which a token amount of free editorial content is thrown up like latticework over a foundation of hard-core photos, video clips, and live streaming video. But don't be too quick to judge a site by its cheesy banner ads; you can't always predict where you might find some articulate, sex-savvy personality slinging quips, reviews, and advice. For example, the webmaster for Porno for Monkeys Like You, an annotated directory of hard-core sex sites, promotes a variety of perspectives on his site by sponsoring a thoughtful, woman-produced erotic newsletter called *screech*.

Webmaster Wyyrd of *Hoot Island Graphics* uses his site for two purposes: to promote the "philosophy that Sex Is Fun as opposed to Sex Is Nasty," and to make merciless fun of the conventions of adult pay sites. While he offers some of the same nudie pix you'll find on many other adult sites, he surrounds these with silly erotica, goofy words of wisdom, and hysterical parodies of the ways in which male consumers let themselves get scammed. As he points out, "It's easy to just download a bunch of pictures and put them all online for money without needing to put any thought into it at all, because so much of the audience really doesn't care. If you were to take a cute picture of a dog, call it 'Anne and Cathy's Doggie-Style Page,' and advertise it in a newsgroup, describing it honestly, you'd still have a thousand hits by the end of the day. . . . I love bucking the trend, if for no other reason than that I get to meet so many cool people that way." And in fact, his approach has earned him so many female fans that, by popular request, he now offers nudie pix of men as well.

Content Is Queen

A handful of adult e-zines are full-fledged, deluxe periodicals providing quality content and professional gloss. Some, such as the online editions of *Libido* or *Paramour*, exist primarily for promotion, providing a free preview of the style and content of their print magazines in order to expand their subscriber base. In rare cases, erotic e-zines are attempting to follow the model of trail-blazing Web magazines such as *Salon* by cultivating a stable of established contributors and offering top-notch material for free in hopes of building a readership and advertising base that will eventually prove profitable. They're able to woo both contributors and readers with what *Nerve* magazine's editor Genevieve Field refers to as "a little editorial bravery"—a scarce commodity offline. *Nerve* was launched with an enviable media splash in 1997, and Genevieve notes that "We were able to take a passion for edgy writing and $100,000 and turn it into a magazine that is now being read by hundreds of thousands of people. There is no way we could have done this in print. The costs of promoting, printing, and distributing a magazine on a national level are so high that print magazines have to be very demographically calculated, safe publications. People aren't taking real gut-wrenching risks."

But *Nerve* would never have achieved its high profile if the editors hadn't been committed to building a readership of both women and men. As Genevieve puts it, "*Nerve* is groundbreaking because it has a sizable female audience; women read *Nerve* because they have more sexual agency today than before—because they are willing to indulge more sexual personae, and because they are increasingly bored with erotica and its tired recipes for arousal. We believe (unlike our competitors) that women can be turned on by photography and men can be turned on by original, inventive prose."

Worth a Thousand Words

And those women who *are* turned on by photography can find abundant material online, if they're willing to hack through the jungle of what one fed-up survey respondent so vividly describes as "ads flashing women's asses and pussies in my face—those damn flickering click-me bars with a pussy opening and shutting." Perhaps you've never even tried to find erotic visuals online, assuming that there was nothing out there but what another survey respondent refers to as "typical crotch shots and boring sex poses." Or perhaps you've gone surfing, only to reach the following conclusion: "So far I haven't come up with any sites where the focus is at least half on depicting an attractive man intensely involved with his female partner! Most of the sites with pictures don't seem aware of possible women consumers."

Don't despair! There are actually some gorgeous erotic visual images on the Web that would otherwise be unavailable except in the pages of very expensive coffee-table books or on the walls of alternative art galleries. Sites such as *Nerve* magazine and the Fine Art Nude Photography Network feature photography by some of the most talented artists of the day. On fine-art or fetish sites, you can find photos in which men, as well as women, are subjects of the camera's gaze. However, if you're seeking hard-core imagery of men, you'll probably have to be as persistent and creative as this survey respondent: "I look for smut depicting full frontal male nudity. The traditional porn magazines I've seen either place all the emphasis on the female body or aren't very picky about the attractiveness of the men. I've had more success finding scintillating shots online, especially on gay male sites, which often have pix I enjoy."

Unfortunately, even the alternative erotic photography you'll find on the Web can lack diversity; the majority of the models are white and conform to certain mainstream standards of beauty. For greater variety, look to the wealth of erotic fine arts online. A couple of sites—notably Dr. Susan Block's Erotics Gallery, Ars Magna Erotica, and the World Museum of Erotic Art—provide a fascinating visual history of erotic paintings, sculptures, and decorative arts from around the world. While some of these sites do charge subscription fees, all have sample images on view so you can

WHAT WOMEN WANT

"Anything other than models with hair that drips hair spray, globs of eye shadow, and hideously long chocolate-colored fingernails is welcome, and the models *must* look as though they're enjoying themselves, or what's the point?"

decide whether you want to pay to see the works that weren't included in your high school art history class.

Finally, numerous pay sites offer the visual immediacy of video clips or live streaming video. In live streaming video, real-time sexual performances are transmitted onto your computer screen, and you can direct and interact with the performer(s) by typing commands and comments back and forth. The style and content of this material comes straight out of hard-core video, and it would look a lot better (a lot faster!) on your TV screen. The producers of Herotica, one of the few pay sites geared toward women, argue that "We don't feel that live video appeals to women the same way it appeals to men. In our experience, we have found that cybersex doesn't appeal to women as much as cybervoyeurism does. Images, videostreams, or even video phone calls that involve interfacing with another person are too invasive." Given the increasing women's market for adult videos, and the rising popularity of the video conferencing technology you'll read about in chapter 7, "Online Rendezvous," we're a little suspicious of this assessment. We think women are just choosier consumers who aren't impressed by the high prices and formulaic content of most video streams. After all, we and many of our survey respondents have nothing against hard-core imagery; we just aren't going to sit around watching a jumpy, slow-loading clip of a blow job that fills about three-by-three grainy inches on a computer monitor when we could enjoy an entire video from the comfort of the living-room sofa—and spend a lot less money in the process. As video streaming technology improves, it will be interesting to see whether any innovative webmistresses put together a site designed to appeal to women.

Community Builders

Online sex magazines truly transcend the print medium by bringing people together in communities of shared interest . . . and by creating forums in which they can talk about sex! Online readers of *Hip Mama* (see p. 116) get the same tips and tirades on modern-day parenting available in the print zine, but they enjoy the bonus of discussion boards, which provide access to a limitless pool of parents who are also grappling with topics such as "Sex with the kid in the bed, anyone?" or "Help, I've misplaced my sex drive!" Visitors to *Loving More* can do more than just read up on the philosophy of consensual nonmonogamy; they can drop in on its chat room to discuss what it's really like to put the principles of polyamory into practice.

One of the most exciting manifestations of this culture of more explicit, more accurate sex talk can be found in the chat rooms and message boards of a new breed of women's e-zines. A loosely linked network called

"EstroNet" links "estrogen-powered" Web zines such as *Maxi*, *Bust*, and *Postfeminist Playground*, all of which are helmed by smart, high-energy, twenty-something women who tackle the topics of gender, culture, media, and sex with equal aplomb. We're both over thirty, so we can't pretend to understand the distinctions among grrls, new-order girls, or postfeminists—we just know that all these women sound like they'd be fun to have drinks with. These aren't sex magazines or feminist magazines, per se, but lo and behold, in the message boards and forums of the EstroNet, girls and women are talking about sex in a funny, honest, straight-shooting way that you'd never see reflected in mainstream women's magazine articles such as "Seven Erogenous Zones *You* Should Know About."

We revel in the fact that, thanks to the Web, teenage girls and women in their forties can chat together about their favorite vibrators or read a thoughtful article about female-to-male transsexualism right alongside a paean to nail polish. We love knowing that mothers across the country can tune in to *Hip Mama* for tips on postpartum sex, or that busy career women can take a break from their workdays to tour *Kinky Cards'* photo gallery. After all, as the webmistress of *Venus or Vixen?* puts it, "any porn you can see from the privacy of your home/office/wherever is good porn."

The Web offers a birds-eye view of the wide expanse of sexual possibilities, combined with a culture of total anonymity, full disclosure, and explicit discourse. One of our survey respondents comments that "online entertainment offers almost unlimited freedom of expression, plus the thrill of knowing someone wants you to look and dares you to read all about it." For women willing to accept this dare, the payoff can be a new appreciation of their own authentic desires.

Reviews

EROTICA

CompuServe's Erotica Forum

This popular erotica forum, which welcomes both women and men, is currently limited to CompuServe members (however, they may soon open their Web site to the general public). The forum is located in "Readers' and Writers' Ink," where you'll also find the "Hot Romance" forum, writers' groups, and an extensive archive of contributors' work.

Custom Erotica Source

http://www.customeroticasource.com

Not sure what to get your sweetie on your next anniversary? How about a fourteen-page erotic story starring the two of you! You don't have to be Anaïs Nin to pull this off—the folks at Custom Erotica Source will take your fantasies and turn them into a finely crafted naughty tale (for a fee, of course). You fill out a detailed questionnaire, specifying your preference of language (smutty vs. euphemistic), gender, sexual orientation, and genre (romance, suspense, mystery, etc.), toss in a few sexual details, mail it off, and within twelve days a nicely bound gift will arrive. The company claims that all tales are unique; they don't use fill-in-the-blank templates. Several samples appear online, along with some attractive erotic artwork.

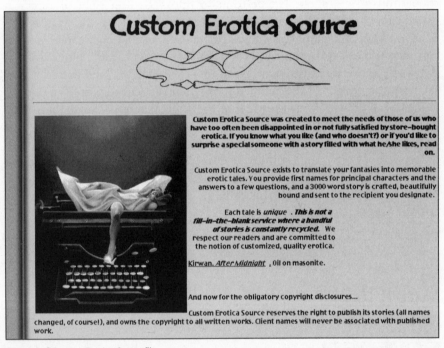

Custom Erotica Source

Custom Erotica Source was created to meet the needs of those of us who have too often been disappointed in or not fully satisfied by store-bought erotica. If you know what you like (and who doesn't?) or if you'd like to surprise a special someone with a story filled with what he/she likes, read on.

Custom Erotica Source exists to translate your fantasies into memorable erotic tales. You provide first names for principal characters and the answers to a few questions, and a 3000 word story is crafted, beautifully bound and sent to the recipient you designate.

Each tale is *unique* . *This is not a fill-in-the-blank service where a handful of stories is constantly recycled.* We respect our readers and are committed to the notion of customized, quality erotica.

Kirwan, *After Midnight* , oil on masonite.

And now for the obligatory copyright disclosures...

Custom Erotica Source reserves the right to publish its stories (all names changed, of course!), and owns the copyright to all written works. Client names will never be associated with published work.

Copyright©Custom Erotica Source™

Dreams Unlimited

http://www.dreams-unlimited.com

If you like romance fiction that's out-of-this-world—literally—you've found the right site. Dreams Unlimited specializes in "otherworldly romance," which means that heroines are more likely to end up in the arms of aliens, ghosts, or vampires than those of handsome strangers. This site was started by a few veteran romance writers who grew tired of the formulaic story lines required by mainstream publishers and chose to electronically self-publish material with an emphasis on fantasy, futuristic, and paranormal plots, as well as gay and lesbian themes. The bulk of the material on this site is romance fiction, but you'll also find a cache of "erotic romance," which the authors describe as follows: "Erotica and Erotic Romance are not the same. Erotica is, by definition, sexually explicit literature, whereas Erotic Romance centers on the relationship and the story, rather than the sexual exploits of the characters. It is still guaranteed to 'Steam your socks off' as one reader put it." Generous excerpts from each book are posted on the site, but you must pay a small fee to order the complete work, which is sent via e-mail or on a disk. A discussion board and special newsletter are available to members (membership is free), and complete writers' guidelines are posted on the site.

Eli's Erotica Archive

http://www.netusa.net/~eli/erotica.html

Eli has compiled a comprehensive archive of erotic fiction from the Usenet groups alt.sex.stories and rec.arts.erotica.

Erotasy

http://www.erotasy.com

Devoted to "extraordinary erotic literature," this San Francisco-based site delivers well-written short stories that will stimulate both your mind and your body. Wide-ranging in style and content, Erotasy's stories are written by notable contemporary erotica writers of all sexualities. Check out the site's expanding free section, which includes an ongoing serial that is updated weekly. The remainder of the stories are for sale; you read an excerpt, then download the story for a nominal fee through the site's secure server.

Erotica Readers Association

http://www.erotica-readers.com

A lovingly tended island in the sea of online erotica, the Erotica Readers Association was created by and for women and men who enjoy dis-cussing, writing, and reading erotica "written with a woman's view of sen-suality." Written erotica is the primary focus of this site, but reviews also cover movies—both R- and X-rated—and music. The ERA serves as an excellent gateway resource for erotica lovers. Visitors to the site are encouraged to subscribe so they can add their two cents about their "favorite sensual scenes" to the ongoing postings. Much of the site consists of reviews and recommendations submitted by site subscribers, whose tastes range from what you might call "hard-core Harlequin" to porn noir. While this means the quality of reviews can vary from crisp and witty to grade-school-book-report, it adds to the chatty, community-based feel of the site—feedback from erotica authors and their fans are posted side by side.

Aspiring writers will appreciate the regularly updated list of author's guidelines for submissions to erotic magazines and publishers. And the directory of recommended Web sites and newsgroups is a boon to anyone who's ever tried to dive into the vast, undifferentiated tangle of Usenet groups devoted to erotica. Instead, you can scroll down this carefully hand-picked list to find referrals to the best sites for erotica on a variety of top-

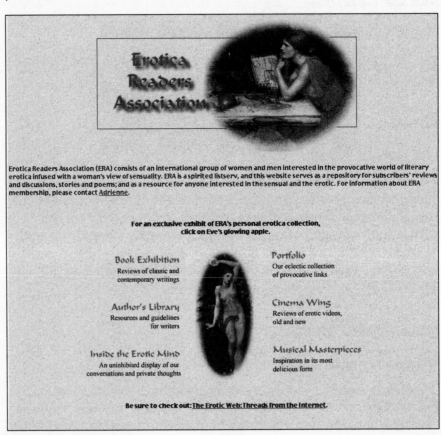

Webmistress: Adrienne Benedicks Images: Sandra Jones and Anne Bulin.

ics—from group sex to science fiction to romance to fetishizing robots. The site links to the online bookstore Amazon.com, so you can order many of the compelling books you read about; and there are links to other online resources as well as a listing of mail-order sources for erotic books and videos.

Erotic Vox—BDSM Erotica

http://www.eroticvox.com

Webmistress Voxana invites readers to partake of "well-written consensual stories that reflect the exchange of power within a BDSM relationship. This means that BOTH parties receive pleasure on levels that are healthy and empowering." She makes good on her promise, delivering plenty of hot fiction (written by herself and other contributors) and updating the site regularly with new material. She also features a separate page with vanilla writings, a chat room, message boards, a bookstore linked to Amazon.com, links to other resources, and a provocative collection of BDSM-related quotes from famous people, such as this one from George Eliot: "There is a sort of subjection which is the peculiar heritage of largeness and of love; and strength is often only another name for willing bondage to irremediable weakness."

Joan Elizabeth Lloyd

http://www.joanlloyd.com

Joan Elizabeth Lloyd writes about sex and fantasies the way a master chef prepares a fine meal—with experience, passion, and a taste for the exotic. This author of several popular erotic novels and self-help books maintains a site that's regularly updated with lots of spicy new material. In addition to posting her erotic fiction, Lloyd writes a Q&A sex column and dispenses monthly tips about sexual enhancement for couples, such as communicating in bed, introducing anal sex, and trying new sexual adventures. She practices what she preaches—she and her husband experimented with a video camera pointed to their bed—and charms readers with her enthusiastic approach to sex. An impressive list of links to sex information and erotica sites rounds out her site. Lloyd is a completely endearing, mischievous cheerleader for erotic expression; you'll find yourself revisiting her site often for inspiration.

Mary Anne's Home Page

http://www.iam.com/maryanne

Mary Anne's writing will arouse, her enthusiasm will inspire, and her tremendous resource listings will inform. Dismayed by the lack of good material online, Mary Anne Mohanraj started posting erotic stories on the Internet in 1992. Today she's got a Web site overflowing with steamy erotica and romantic poetry, a published book of her work, and a faithful fan club. Her extensive writers' resource section makes Mary Anne's site one of the most useful stops for those interested in writing or publishing erotica. The highlights include an exhaustive listing of magazine and book publishers, articles about how to write erotica, legal explanations of copyright issues, interviews with popular online erotica authors, and an online erotica writing workshop. Mary Anne also reprints columns she's written for other magazines on a variety of sexual topics. She includes good, selective links to other sex sites and rounds out her site by sharing her other hobbies: fans of science fiction and fantasy literature will appreciate her annotated bibliographies (including one for kids' books), and entrepreneurs can learn how to create their own Web pages.

The Pink Kink Catalog

http://www.razberry.com/raz/pink/top.htm

Canadian journalist Donna Laframboise's "catalog" sells a concept, not a product—she's collected sexually explicit excerpts from romance novels to illustrate her thesis that these books are the female answer to *Penthouse*. Those who've never sampled the romance genre may be surprised to discover that male bondage and sex toy use are depicted right along with passionate kisses and melting glances. She includes a compelling introduction about how antiporn feminists turn a blind eye to what is clearly an insatiable female need for textual pornography, noting that romance novels are an almost billion-dollar-a-year business and are "an important element of 'female culture' whose contents have remained a dirty little secret for far too long."

Q*ink! A Lesbian and Gay Writing Community

http://users.lanminds.com/~pherrin28

A fantastic resource for gay and lesbian writers, Q*ink! boasts one of the most well-maintained "call for submissions" sections—including a page devoted to erotica—that we've encountered online, along with helpful links to agents, editorial services, and writing groups. A calendar of events (most of which occur in San Francisco) is also updated regularly. Members post individual pages with biographical information and excerpts from their work.

Straight Women's Erotica

http://womenserotica.miningco.com

Tired of Harlequins that leave you hanging? Too embarrassed to buy a *Playgirl?* Relief awaits you on this playful, upbeat site, comprised mainly of links hand-picked by Holly O'Neill, one of the reviewers for the online directory The Mining Company. The site focuses on material geared toward heterosexual women and boasts an impressive array of annotated links to sites with written erotica and nude male photos, as well as masturbation-related and hard-core sites. You'll also find erotica submitted by visitors, sex tips from Holly, and a discussion board. An excellent starting point for women interested in exploring a variety of online erotica.

Wild Women Dreamin' Wet

http://dykesworld.de

Drop in on some steamy lesbian locker-room sex or a lusty voyeur's tryst with her twin sister's lover. These are some of the tales dreamed up by the wild women who contribute their erotic stories and poems to this friendly and inviting site. You'll find an impressive variety of characters indulging in vanilla and S/M sex, obsessing over lost loves, engaging in May/December romances, running afoul of the law, and generating lots and lots of heat. Currently there are close to one hundred stories, but new material is posted every few days, so this number should grow exponentially. Minimal graphics ensure that the stories pop up quickly, but the site does include some erotic photographs and illustrations placed within the text to please the eye. Women from around the world contribute (and provide entertaining short bios), and a few stories appear in German. Anyone can get a story posted, so the quality of the writing runs the gamut, and occasional typos and formatting snafus can be distracting. Apparently, these wild women have received some hate mail, which the site administrators creatively counter by posting these ridiculous tirades along with their own snappy comebacks.

FAN FICTION

Slash Fan Fiction WebRing Homepage

http://www.geocities.com/SoHo/Cafe/3040/slash.html

A rapidly-growing Web ring connecting over one hundred sites specializing in slash fiction.

Yahoo's Fan Fiction Directory

http://www.yahoo.com/news_and_media/television/fan_fiction

From "The Adventures of Sinbad" to "The X-Files," you'll find hundreds of conveniently categorized sites devoted to fan fiction.

The Xenaverse Codex: The bardeyes & xenabat Library

http://www.xenafiction.net

Xena stars in our own fantasies, so we couldn't resist adding this site, which boasts writings by over five hundred authors and focuses on a lesbian relationship between the TV show's heroines, Xena and Gabrielle.

FEMALE EROTICA AUTHORS' HOMEPAGES

Angela Preston (site name: X-Stories)

http://www.xstories.com

Anne's Erotic Story Archives

http://annejet.pair.com

The Erotic Mind of Emma Holly

http://www2.wavetech.net/~emmah/eroticmind

Sabrina's Erotica

http://www.sabrina.org

Vivienne LaFay (site name: Erotica Femina)

http://www.elated.com/erotica-femina

ART AND PHOTOGRAPHY

Ars Magna Erotica

http://www.azstarnet.com/~nik/AME

Hundreds of erotic images are reproduced on this site, lovingly constructed by a Swedish engineering student. A timeline of erotica allows viewers to pick and choose from a wide range of primarily Western genres and artists, a nice feature when you're not sure what will strike your fancy: Pornographic Greek pottery? Sexual symbolism in surrealist paintings? Bawdy eighteenth-century caricatures? Images can also be viewed chronologically, accompanied by a somewhat canned art history lesson. A few contemporary photographers are featured, along with links to other sites related to their work.

While the exquisite images earn this site high marks, the accompanying text is somewhat sophomoric. Fortunately, there's not much of it. When the author sticks to reciting facts and dates, he's simply pedestrian, but when he theorizes about the distinctions between art and pornography or abuses words like *vulgar* and *deviant,* he's downright annoying. This is the effort of a loving amateur, not Kenneth Clark (or even Sister Wendy), so don't expect scrupulous accuracy; a section entitled "Ancient Paintings" offers no approximate dates, locations, or names of artists and contains Victorian artwork. You can expect the images to come up quickly and vividly at about one-quarter-screen size—an option to view them full-screen would be the icing on the cake.

Auto Erotic House of Art

http://www.netlabs.net/hp/jimr/art/flash.html

Even the shyest would-be-exhibitionist would be hard-pressed to resist the come-on of artist Pez Bono's unique site. "Amateurs, send in your washed out, bent up, grainy, dusty, unfocused, flashburned, dirty lensed, yellowcast, thumb in the picture home shots and see them turned into fabulous works of art." Through digital manipulation (including filtering, color adjustments, and abstracting the background), Pez transforms ordinary Kodak moments into art pieces that resemble silk-screens or David Hockney paintings. And he'll give you a digital nip and tuck wherever you request. All he asks in return is permission to display finished pieces on his site. So what have you got to lose? New soft-core pix of both men and women are added every few days. Though Pez has plans to add a subscription hard-core section, he comments in an interview on Jane Duvall's site that "my site's more about expression and boosting people's confidence in their own desirability than any kind of voyeuristic arousal."

Erotic Muse

http://www.eroticmuse.com

This ambitious pay site promotes itself as offering "the very best in erotica from around the world for discerning individuals," and indeed, its collection of erotic images is impressive both in quantity and quality. You'll find fine art reproductions, art from "erogenous zones of history," a bit of a hodgepodge of contemporary photography, and—most notably—a cinema section featuring clips of classic stag films from 1910 to 1946. The limited written content on the site includes some rather highfalutin literary excerpts such as Greek epigrams. Alas, the site currently suffers from techno-overload: sound files make it slow to load, and because of its excessive use of frames, images are restricted to one-third-screen size. Still, Erotic Muse merits a look, as guests have access to a generous helping of sample images. An online store offers rare books and collectibles.

Erotics Gallery

http://www.eroticsgallery.com

A dream of a site for browsing, the Erotics Gallery is the online version of a small private gallery in New York City. With a focus on the past hundred years of erotic art, the gallery includes works of all media and from a wide range of countries: European prints, Japanese woodblock prints, Chinese porcelains, contemporary American paintings, Indian miniature watercolors on ivory, and even World War II pin-up cards. Brief, informational descriptions enhance, rather than intrude on, your viewing pleasure. All of the art depicted is for sale. Prices range from ten dollars for posters up to several thousand dollars for one-of-a-kind antiques. There's no question that you can spend a highly enjoyable, instructive couple of hours reviewing the wares. The site is a bit slow to load; the reproductions are on the small side (most are less than one-quarter screen, with a few at half screen) but of good quality.

Eroto~

http://www.eroto.com

We can't praise the artistic and technical quality of this virtual fine-art gallery highly enough. The artist in residence is R. C. Hörsch, and the site is primarily devoted to a revolving exhibition of erotic photography spanning his thirty-year career. Plans are under way to add exhibit space for other notables of erotic photography, such as Charles Gatewood and Michael Rosen.

In an interesting approach to content issues, all visitors are expected to set their own limits by selecting their comfort levels (none, mild, moderate, and extreme) with regard to violence, politics, nudity, and eroticism. As is courteously noted, "If your preferences are set to 'none' you will see very little artwork on this site!" Extreme violence is defined as including realistic depictions of pain, gore, death, and dismemberment, but these are art shots by and large, and whether a representation of a nude woman posed on a cross is disturbing or thought-provoking is in the eye of the viewer. Guests can view a handful of free samples, while members have access to page after page of "pansexual" photographs. Images load swiftly in thumbnail size, with up to ten images per page. You have the option of selecting a full-screen view of all photos and a detail view of many. Most photos are black and white. (As Hörsch notes slyly in the interview posted on this site, "I've heard it said that if you shoot in black and white it's art, but that if you shoot in color it's pornography. I do both.") Gallery-quality prints and copies of Hörsch's video documentary series, *Lovers: An Intimate Portrait*, are for sale through a secure server.

Fine Art Nude Photography Network

http://www.fineartnude.com/webring

This Web ring links thirty sites featuring the finest fine-art nude photography in a wide range of styles: black-and-white, infrared, and Polaroid image-transfer. You can view samples of each artist's work on the Web ring's home page, then visit the sites you choose. The photographers represented here—and their subjects—are both male and female (though, as in nude art down through the ages, female subjects predominate).

Gut Art Gallery

http://www.gutart.rit.se

Swedish artist Heinz Guth devotes much of the space in his online gallery to his exuberant paintings, sketches, and watercolors of "BBWs," or big beautiful women, along with a range of fine-art nudes, both male and female. He also provides links to other BBW art sites.

Herotica: Erotica for Women

http://www.her-erotica.com

If you bemoan the lack of sexual entertainment for women online, you must visit this site created by a group of women who had the same beef. They've produced a beautiful, tasteful, and sexy gallery filled with visual and written erotica for women, which comes at a modest price. Subscribers to Herotica will gain access to a large cache of erotic art, from delectable vin-

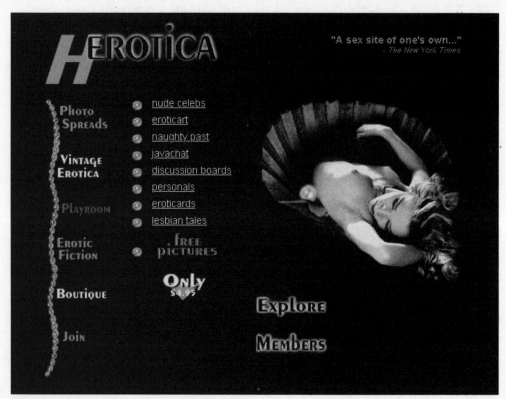

Copyright©Spiral Designs

tage images of pin-ups and daguerreotype boudoir shots to dazzling contemporary photos of male and female nudes, lesbian sex, and fetish fashion. When you've had enough of the highbrow images, indulge your tabloid tastes by viewing the slide show of nude stars. Whether you prefer full frontals of Brad Pitt and Mel Gibson or the bare breasts of Demi Moore and Susan Sarandon, inquiring minds won't be disappointed. The images load first as thumbnails, to save time, and you select those you'd like to view full-screen. If the written word does more for your libido, partake of the site's many lesbian tales or contribute to an ongoing erotic novel. Post a message on Herotica's discussion board, visit the chat room, or check out the free personals. You can take a free tour of the site before subscribing, but there are only a handful of free samples. Herotica connects to a free nonexplicit women's site called HerSalon. The banner ads here aren't too intrusive and usually steer you to other interesting women's sites.

Isle of Lesbos: Lesbian Images in Art

http://www.sappho.com

"A place of art, culture and learning for women-oriented women," Isle of Lesbos features lesbian-themed poetry and art that's in the public domain, along with a nice collection of quotes attributed to sapphic notables from Natalie Barney to Two Nice Girls. The poetry section includes a biography, a list of selected works, and an assortment of Web and print reference materials on each poet. The art section features close to one hundred works dating from 1500 to 1935, selected for their portrayal of "romantic or emotional interaction between women, not all sexual." You can view the images as either thumbnails or gorgeous full-screen reproductions.

Kinky Cards

http://www.kinkycards.com

Whether you're commemorating Valentine's Day, National Masturbation Day, or a private anniversary, there's bound to be an electronic greeting card in the well-stocked galleries of Kinky Cards that's an appropriate expression of your sentiments. Art and photography from all eras and all styles—both subtly sensuous and flagrantly fetishistic—are available here for free. This site is maintained by the couple behind the excellent resource site Ds Kiosk (see p. 190) and features work by some of the premier erotic and fetish photographers of our day.

Matt's Party Page (formerly Party Dancer Online)

http://www.wenet.net/~mwelsh/party

In the mood for some wholesome beefcake? Tired of fishing in gay male waters? Head over to *Playgirl* model Matt Welsh's homepage and treat yourself to a peek at the washboard abs of this honest-to-God nice guy. Matt's a software engineer who's starting a family with his wife, Maria (check out the sonogram pix of their firstborn). He first went online to advertise his availability as a dancer for bachelorette parties (that's how he paid his way through school), but his photos proved to be such a hit that he began moonlighting as a nude model—you'll find a rotating archive of photos at this site, which Matt no longer updates. If you're tired of envelope-pushing pix of fetish scenes and radical sex, Matt's tasteful "Adonis-on-the-beach" shots just might float your boat.

Michael Rosen

http://www.shaynew.com

Michael Rosen has been photographing the radical sex scene in the San Francisco Bay Area since the early '80s. On his small but compelling site you'll find a selection of photos from all three of his self-published books, as well as works in progress. From cinema verité photos that will take you right into the heat of an S/M encounter to studio portraits exploring gender play and body modification, Rosen's photos are elegant, explicit, erotic, and utterly unique. Photos load quickly at anywhere from one-quarter- to half-screen size.

Lee Stranahan's Erotica

http://www.stranahan.com/erotica

A producer of what he calls "digital fine-art pornography," Lee Stranahan works in collaboration with his models (all amateurs) to explore and express their sexual fantasies. Most of the lush, black-and-white photos in this well-stocked gallery are of women, and many have fetish or S/M themes. Thumbnails load quickly to half-screen size. There's a nice, unpretentious feel to this free site; the artist includes information about his work with his wife, along with an excellent, annotated set of links to other art sites, other erotic photographers, and sex pioneers he admires.

World Museum of Erotic Art

http://www.opkamer.nl/amea/index.shtml

This online museum was founded by a group of Dutch artists, who note, "Although much of the material here is considered pornographic in many countries, it is the strong belief of the founders that looking at imagery concerning the act of love will do no damage to your health." Guests can send free electronic erotic postcards, visit the site's message boards (probably among the few online with subject headers such as "Homoerotic Anime" or "Architecture and Eroticism"), and tour the current free exhibit on a theme such as "machinery" or "Japanese prints." Members (and anyone who signs up for a free trial membership) have access to a wide-ranging collection of predominantly European historical and contemporary art. Thumbnails load quickly, and reproductions are displayed full-screen. Our only caveat about this site would be its goofy, and occasionally tasteless, captions.

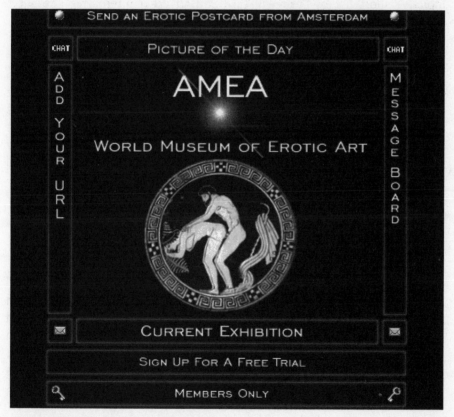

Copyright©AMEA/World Museum of Erotic Art

Anything That Moves

http://www.anythingthatmoves.com

This well-designed Web site offers choice excerpts from the print zine *Anything That Moves*, which is published three times a year. You can review the offerings issue-by-issue or select from general categories: articles, erotic poetry and fiction, book reviews, resources, and quirky entertainment, including an advice column and the "Dear Jane" soap opera, written round-robin by staff and friends. The writing here is friendly and engaging, and the articles tackle unusual topics such as how to find a bi-friendly therapist, the history of the educational performance group the Safer Sex Sluts, how intersex births are handled in the United States, and more. A short list of links will take you to other alternative sexuality sites.

Bodice

http://www.bodice.com

Editors Gizelle and Zoe, self-described "femmes extraordinaire," launched this e-zine dedicated to women's health and sexuality in response to their observation that most magazines on the newsstands are geared "toward teenage airheads, aspiring super-models or craft-crazed suburbanites. There is little available for real, live women with real world needs." Gizelle and Zoe come across as New Age Helen Gurly Browns, and *Bodice* is definitely an e-zine for women, not grrls. Tips on plastic surgery, aphrodisiacs, and seducing married men are sprinkled in among sex advice, book reviews, and erotic anecdotes. Astrology and aromatherapy (*Bodice* promises to launch its own line of products) provide the New Age content.

We enjoy the high spirits and sex-positive spin of this zine. It's also a treat to read an online magazine geared toward women over thirty. Our only major quibble is with the awkward organization. *Bodice* suffers mightily from the cutesy-header syndrome: it's pretty much impossible to tell whether editorial content will be stashed in the "Boudoir" section or the "Hot Bodice" section. And who could guess that the astrology column is filed under "Eat, Drink and Be Merry"?

Brat Attack

http://www.devildog.com/brat

The print version of *Brat Attack*, "the zine for leatherdykes and other bad girls," shot briefly across the San Francisco horizon between 1991 and 1994. With its take-no-prisoners irreverence, a refreshing willingness to give equal time to exposing sexual biases within and without the leather community, and an impressive range of topics, *Brat Attack* stood out from the pack. All issues of the print zine are sold out, but editor and graphic artist Fish has posted the text of *Brat Attack*'s articles on her Web site for posterity. Anyone's sexual horizons will benefit from the assumption-busting influence of articles and transcripts of round-table discussions on leathersex, gender play, butch identity, transsexualism, class issues, and more. The site includes a handful of links to related online zines and S/M resources.

Bust

http://www.bust.com

For women who like to dish the dirt (and who doesn't?), this magazine's for you. *Bust* bills itself as "the voice of the New Order Girl" but could just as easily be the voice of "chicks with attitude." Part of the EstroNet brigade of "estrogen-powered" online zines, *Bust* offers a lively, humorous, savvy review of gender issues, media, and culture. Although not a sex magazine, *Bust* regularly expresses an attitude of sexual entitlement and appreciation that's heady stuff. Take this priceless excerpt from "Dixie LaRue's" 1997 article about blow jobs: "As adult sexual politics became more apparent, so too did my predilection for cock-suckage. It was one of the few times a girl could feel as though she were making an impression. Usually my friends and I just felt, well, used. Sucking cock, you felt important. No longer acted upon, above or below the waist, now you were the actor, the doer instead of the 'do-ee,' or worse, the 'done-to.' For once, you had the upperhand. Fellatio put you in the driver's seat."

The author goes on to enumerate her fellatio "pet peeves," and you can bet the next time you've got your head in some guy's lap you're going to remember this piece and laugh out loud. It would be tempting to target the audience for this magazine as Gen-X girls, but that would be selling it short. Whether the issue is devoted to sex, goddesses, crushes, or parenthood, there's something in it for opinionated women of all ages. Sadly, only a handful of articles from the paper zine appear online—but with a clean, witty presentation, links to a slew of women's sites, active conference sites, and "live chick chat," the online *Bust* is clearly more a community clearinghouse than a publication.

Future Sex

http://www.futuresex.com

The online survivor of one of the '90s most ambitious erotic print magazines, *Future Sex* offers unbeatable erotic images from fine photographers such as Craig Morey, Ralph Steinmeier, and Phyllis Christopher. Archived photos and drawings load quickly at full-screen size. Several different artists are featured in each issue, and readers are encouraged to submit their own science fiction fantasy art—see, for example, Asia Carerra's line drawings of Amazonian babes with wasp waists. The remainder of the site consists of science fiction and fantasy erotica, primarily written by men. Again, reader contributions are welcome. While *Future Sex* has ambitions of appealing equally to women and men, its links and banner ads lean heavily toward porno pay sites ("Asian girls with shaven pussies"), which female readers may find distracting at best. Plans are in the works to add advice columns, chat rooms, and interactive opportunities galore.

Gray Areas

http://www.grayarea.com

"In life there is no black and white, only Gray Areas," state the editors of this online version of a paper zine dedicated to subject matter that is "illegal, immoral and/or controversial." Encompassing alternative, lifestyles and subcultures of every variety, *Gray Areas'* subject matter includes computers and technology (think hackers); drugs (from acid to plasma); law and criminal justice (what goes on behind bars); music (the editors are unabashed Deadheads); and sex. Editor Netta Gilboa has a background in journalism, women's studies, and sociology, with a specialty in criminal deviance. As she notes, "it's not every sex researcher who can befriend both porn stars and antiporn crusaders." Each issue features at least one sex or adult-industry-related article or interview, and the editors display a well-informed respect for the adult industry that is all too rare in a lefty zine. If for no other reason, we recommend visiting the site to check out its excellent, wide-ranging interview with feminist adult filmmaker Candida Royalle.

Material from the paper zine is not particularly recent, but the site itself is updated regularly. The editors issue their own "Gray Areas on the Web" awards monthly to honor unusual Web sites, with subject matter ranging from Asia Carerra to voodoo. Check out the extensive and up-to-date links for all the zine's major topics, as well as reviews of books, zines, catalogs, video games, software, CD-ROMs, and movies.

Hoot Island Graphics

http://www.hootisland.com

Hoot Island is dedicated to the belief that sex can be funny *and* erotic, and that the best sex is often both. The perfect antidote to anyone who has scrolled past one too many banner ads promising "hot teen angels," *Hoot Island* delivers a hysterical parody of pay sites with the "CyberSpooge!" page, which claims to offer "only the finest in borrowed copyrighted images! . . . Why pay some other sleazy, fly-by-night company for pictures you could download for free yourself when you could be paying us instead?"

Webmaster Wyyrd is a thorough, and thoroughly silly, evangelist for the philosophy that sex is funny, not just fun. His "Wacky Wimmin" page links exclusively to R-rated photos of happy, giggling naked women (and a few men to boot)—no sultry, pouting babes allowed. These photos, along with most of the site, are free; in order to view the X-rated photos in the "Hootcore" section, you'll need to sign up with Adult Check (an age-verification service that provides access to thousands of adult sites for an annual fee).

Ranging from the witty to the supremely silly, the "EroticHA" section includes the inspired Hoot Island Interviews with luminaries such as Geneva Daniel of *screech*, erotic graphic artist Phil Foglio, and Asia Carrera, the official patron saint of *Hoot Island*. Submit your true-life tale of something funny that happened to you during sex, read the screenplay for an X-rated *X-Files* episode, and enjoy whatever other nutty takeoffs Wyyrd has posted lately, from Dr. Seuss poems to *Penthouse* letters. The "Pen Squeezins'" page features links to erotic graphic artists such as Phil Foglio, Omaha, and Olivia de Berardinis. And take a moment to appreciate the fact that Wyyrd thoughtfully stashes all banner ads in the "Tourist Trap" page, so they won't intrude on your tour.

Libido: The Journal of Sex and Sensibility

http://www.sensualsource.com/libido

Alone voice of elegant eroticism in the wilderness of skin mags, the print version of *Libido*—"the literary answer to the horizontal urge"—has inspired countless loyal, grateful fans since its inception in 1988. *Libido* specializes in sophisticated erotic stories, lush photographs, illustrations, reviews of books and videos, and even decent poetry. Best of all, subject matter is not limited in any way, and all sexualities are represented with equal élan.

The online *Libido* is currently housed on the SensualSource shopping site (see p. 142), where you can enjoy the current issue of this quarterly and archives of previous issues. *Libido*'s editors also curate SensualSource's free "Fantasy Photo Gallery," which features the cream of the crop of contemporary erotic photography. If you crave European-style nudes, depicting moods that range from sentimental to kinky, you'll want to bookmark this site. Beautifully reproduced works from close to twenty photographers load quickly in thumbnails; unfortunately, due to the frame-happy format of the SensualSource site, most full-size images exceed the limits of the screen. A "Public Gallery" includes amateur photos submitted by exhibitionist readers.

Loving More

http://www.lovemore.com

Whether you're simply curious about or deeply committed to nontraditional relationships, you'll benefit from a visit to this site. *Loving More*, based on a print magazine of the same name, is dedicated to responsible non-monogamy or polyamory: "all forms of multi-partner relating between adults which are ethical and consensual." Only a handful of articles from the magazine are posted (along with subscription information for the print version); the site is primarily designed as a community resource. You'll find information on upcoming conferences, opportunities to order relevant books and back issues of the magazine online, e-mail discussion groups, a chat room, free personals, and a good selection of links to sex-related sites and resources. This is a lifestyle publication, with all the sincerity and occasional cloyingness that a single point of view can entail. Check out the photo of editors Ryam Nearing and Brett Hill, members of a "five-person polyfamily" and their baby boy, born in 1996.

Maxi

http://www.maximag.com

The zine formerly known as *Bitch* and the force behind EstroNet, *Maxi* is a feisty blend of shrewd pop culture commentary and good old-fashioned ranting. Beautifully laid out and easy to navigate, *Maxi* features content that changes weekly, with new themes launched every couple of months (body image, girlfriends, technology). The women of *Maxi* dish up short, snappy articles on gender, media, and culture. And sex, while not the focus of the magazine, is never short-changed. We love the discussion boards that end every article, bringing together girls and women from their teens to their forties to talk about everything from contraception to the Spice Girls to e-mail romance to vibrator tales. All the forums are archived.

mouth organ

http://www.mouthorgan.com

If you enjoy dinner party conversation that is opinionated, outspoken, and good-humored; if you appreciate a spirited argument with anyone who has a wide-ranging intellect, a penchant for sweeping declarations, and an equal willingness to back down and consider your point of view; if you could happily chat about sex, gender, and culture until the wee hours . . . have we got a site for you.

Todd and Debby, the charming, argumentative editors and authors of mouth organ are welcome at either of our dinner tables any time, and their site—which consists of one new essay a week on some subject related to sex, gender, culture, and the Internet—is a favorite with sex neterati such as Mary Anne Mohanraj and Jane of Jane's Net Sex Guide (see p. 192). But we don't mean to imply that you need to be particularly sex- or Internet-savvy to enjoy this site; all that is required is that you enjoy reading a good, thoughtful rant every so often and have an open mind. Past essays, all archived, include "Is the Net Hostile to Women?" and "Net Sex and Courtly Love." The site also offers a user-friendly message board—so you can share your comments with the editors and other readers—and a quirky collection of links and book recommendations.

Nerve

http://www.nerve.com

Frequently praised by our survey respondents, this self-described periodical of "literate smut" is the brainchild of two twenty-something editors whose goal is to provide a "fearless, intelligent forum for both genders" to explore sexual literature, images, and politics. In style and content, Nerve can be a bit too clever for its own good—the counterintuitive layout is a prime example (who could guess that clicking on a globe will take you to the Table of Contents, or that clicking on a ball of yarn will call up "Threads," meaning erotica?). However, the erotic stories and photos are both professional and provocative, and the "Nerve VoiceBox" features interesting and ambitious themed discussions among writers. Nerve accepts submissions only from published authors and exhibited photographers; its wide-ranging contributors list includes Norman Mailer, Al Goldstein, and Daphne Merkin. The work of contemporary artists such as Charles Gatewood and Andres Serrano is particularly stunning. Thumbnails load quickly and full-sized images are about half-screen. The site also features an extensive links listing of sex, health, and literary sites, a boutique, members-only moderated discussion boards, and chat rooms. *Nerve* is translated into German and hosted by the online *Stern* magazine.

Paramour Magazine

http://www.paramour.com

Like its predecessor *Libido*, *Paramour* brings a welcome intelligence to the fine art of erotic literature without sacrificing any heat. *Paramour's* short stories, poetry, and photography embrace all sex styles and levels of kink, and many of the stories go on to be anthologized in print series such as *Best American Erotica*. This online incarnation of the semi-annual print magazine features a sampling of fiction, poetry, book reviews, and photos (illustrating each story) designed to inspire subscriptions. While infrequently updated, this site is a reliable source of steamy, cutting-edge "literary and artistic erotica." Editor Amelia Copeland has also compiled an excellent short list of sex-related links.

Post Feminist Playground

http://www.pfplayground.com

The *Playground* bills itself as a post-modern haven where "boys can be boys, girls can be girls, and everybody has a fun time. Here, the smart girls wear short skirts, the tough boys don't cry, and nobody has to apologize for that." While we're not all that clear about what postfeminism is (are short skirts mandatory?), we heartily recommend the high-energy, tongue-in-cheek writing in this e-zine, another member of EstroNet. Once a month, four "glamatrons" (cartoon vixens named Veronica, Max, Heather, and Pearl, who come complete with bios of their turn-ons and turnoffs) edit articles on the topics of sex, the arts, pop culture, and technology. If you're inspired to comment on what you read, head over to each glamatron's message board, or check out the site's chat room. Veronica's archives are filled with sex-positive rants on topics such as amateur videos, how to deliver successful phone sex, and men faking orgasm.

Salon

http://www.salonmagazine.com

Justifiably hailed as the best-written online magazine, *Salon* makes it onto just about every top-ten Web sites list. But we're not including *Salon* here in the spirit of lemminglike convention; we're including it because *Salon* just happens to feature some of the best sex journalism around. Along with news, reviews, and media analysis, *Salon* routinely tackles topics related to sexual culture, politics, and entertainment in a tone that's blessedly free of the nudge-nudge prurience or aren't we-slumming-now archness that make slogging through mainstream magazines such a chore for anyone with the slightest sexual literacy. Think the magazine's healthy approach to sex has something to do with its home base in San Francisco? We do.

Weekly columns from sex-positive luminaries such as Sallie Tisdale, Susie Bright, and Camille Paglia offer intelligent, provocative entertainment. And don't miss the daily "21st Culture" features for insightful rants about technology and online culture. *Salon*'s format is a model of restraint: easy to read and navigate, judiciously sprinkled with relevant links, well archived, and topped off with a variety of moderated forums in the "Table Talk" section.

Sauce*box

http://www.guillermobosch.com/saucebox/sb.html

*Sauce*box* is that rare, perhaps unique, find—a literary journal utterly lacking in pretension and attitude. Submissions of "well-written, edgy raw passion" are welcome from women and men of all persuasions, and the funny, free-form erotic stories of founding editor T. L. Kelly (a.k.a. Wenchpoet) are among the highlights. In general, the site's stories, reviews, and essays are of a higher caliber than its poetry. *Sauce*box* is blissfully simple in design; the cover page of each issue includes the first paragraphs of each article or piece, so you can browse through all the offerings before clicking on your selection. Contributors to *Sauce*box* seem to belong to a close-knit community, and readers are encouraged to submit e-mail critiques to individual authors. All previous editions of this quarterly are archived on the site.

Scarlet Letters

http://www.scarletletters.com

This bimonthly literary journal of "femmerotica" benefits from quality erotic writing and general high spirits. As editrix Heather Corinna notes in the premiere editorial, "Sharing someone else's arousal is arousing, is it not? What you'll find in *Scarlet Letters* is the work of women kind and bold enough to share, and I'll give you a juicy tidbit, too. I can only speak for myself, but painting and writing about my own arousal is arousing for me in itself. So don't get the idea this is entirely a philanthropic endeavor."

The all-female staff dishes up erotica, nonexplicit art (photos and drawings), poetry, excellent editorial rants (including a no-holds-barred celebration of condoms entitled "For the Love of Latex"), and an advice column, "Ask Mz Scarlet." Heather Corinna is a self-described "tantric Buddhist witch," and *Scarlet Letters*'s content exhibits an appreciation of the sacredness of sex, without being doctrinaire or woo-woo. The short links list includes shopping and safer-sex resources.

Screech

http://pfmly.com/pfmly/screech

Geneva Daniel is the "monkeygirl" behind this endearing zine. Simple in format, each issue of *screech* features one essay courtesy of Geneva, one erotic story, and one true story. Readers are encouraged to submit their own original erotic fiction or true-life tales for posting. And breaking with the online tradition of naked babes, *screech* features a monthly "Hunky Monkey," either photos or a profile of an online dude who has captured Geneva's eye. Archives contain fiction from back issues as well as the archives of Adriana's List, an online erotica forum. Geneva includes a short but solid list of links.

Venus or Vixen?

http://www.venusorvixen.com

A labor of love by an anonymous webmistress, this erotic newsletter is updated weekly. Each issue contains her erotic stories in the "Myths of Venus" section; an essay such as "Tips for Talking Dirty" or a paean to the "Technosexual Revolution"; and erotic art, mostly collages of photos and drawings rather than hard-core images (the webmistress says her mom has helped with some of the artwork). Readers are encouraged to submit contributions, including installments of the site's ongoing erotic story. The sincerity and enthusiasm behind this site are infectious, as evidenced by this editorial excerpt: "I just wanted to say Thank You to the women who have made a difference in sexuality for women. Every woman is invited to grab cord and pull, the second sexual revolution is going to be a long and bumpy ride, but worth every goddamn minute."

Screech is a somewhat erratically published, no-frills erotic e-zine that has earned a legion of fans across the Web largely because of the straight-shooting, humorous writing of editor Geneva Daniel. Okay, the "Hunky Monkey" segment, in which she posts photos of attractive naked men (she has plans to launch a Hunky Monkey gallery), doesn't hurt her site's popularity either. We asked Geneva how a corporate manager and mother of a teenager got started writing and posting her editorials and erotica about sex on the World Wide Web.

"Writing about sex has been an experiment on my part. I always thought I'd enjoy writing as a hobby; why not write about something I like? I think of *screech* as my little writers workshop on the Web. Also, I'm a bit of an exhibitionist. The Web is a magnet for people like me.

"The idea came up during a visit to a friend while reading a column by Isadora Alman in the *New Haven Advocate*. We were having a giggly chick-fest, and we were rolling on the floor laughing over her reply to a reader concerning his ability to insert his penis into his own ass. I thought it might be fun to do something similar on the Web and approached a friend who maintains a porn link/review site for hosting and he loved the idea."

The site has evolved into an e-zine, rather than a Q&A column, and Geneva now publishes her own editorials and erotica, as well as uncensored true-life tales and erotica submitted by readers. Her editorials range all over the map, from a piece arguing that penis size isn't that important (women readers wrote in to agree, men to disagree!) to sex-toy reviews to a lovely piece entitled "Teach Your Children," in which she pays tribute to her parents for communicating their sex-positive attitudes. She gets a lot of mail from readers, a slight majority of whom are men: "Women write mainly to say hello and often to say it's nice to find an adult site with a personal touch. Men write to say how turned on they were by a particular piece. I find that interesting because I had assumed that men would be much more interested in visual stimulation. I also think I have the most interesting collection of really polite 'wanna fuck' letters ever collected."

More and more women like Geneva are going online to explore their thoughts about sex and to provide the erotic entertainment that's been in such short supply until now. Of course, she doesn't fit the stereotype you might have of Sex Sirens in Cyberspace, and she describes the reactions she inspires with typically brisk humor: "The thing that I like the most is probably when I tell someone that I have a silly little sex site on the Web. The facial expressions one gets . . . It's also the thing I like the least sometime, because most people assume I've got to be hanging my boobs and pubes out there for the world to see, and that scares some of them. What frightens me is that automatic negative reaction. What? These people don't fuck? Excuse me . . . make love."

While Geneva launched her site on a lark, she acknowledges that she could "easily give half of my working week to *screech* and love every minute of it. It would be very gratifying to be able to make a living in the adult arena." And gratifying to the rest of us to see the Web filled with sites helmed by smart, sexy women like her.

Wasteland—The Darker Side of Desire

http://www.wasteland.com

An opulent BDSM fetish club and magazine, *Wasteland* delivers top-notch visuals, explicit S/M fiction, informational articles, an international guide to BDSM resources, and a chat room. From Bettie Page to Japanese rope bondage to "pony girls" harnessed to carriages, this site's stock-in-trade is images of beautiful female models—often engaged in scenarios that are off-limits in American porn, such as water sports, extreme S/M, fisting, and penetration with bondage. Needless to say, this material does not come free, but sample images give you a sense of the content. Best of all, this high-gloss site is completely free of banner ads, which only enhances its luxurious appearance.

WHAP! Magazine: Women Who Administer Punishment

http://www.whapmag.com

"The modern woman's guidebook to marital bliss," *WHAP!* is a hysterically funny pastiche of 1950s women's magazines . . . with a twist. This quarterly magazine "brings you the advice, support and know-how you need to run your household with a firm hand, from the kitchen all the way upstairs to your bedroom." Every issue includes a "Punishment Assignment," so in no time you'll have learned what "you need to know to make your man please you—not the other way around!"

Alas, there isn't much magazine content online, but do check out this site, if only to read the scathingly funny FAQ section, entitled "Spankbait: Our Most Frequently Asked Stupid Questions," in which the editors make merciless fun of the gents who write in with sexual solicitations. You'll also find a weekly online advice column, an excellent list of links to other femdom resources, and the Retro Systems online catalog, from which you can order subscriptions, back issues of the magazine, femdom publications, videos, and "maternal discipline tools," such as the WHAP! hairbrush, "sissy panties," and strap-on. Online ordering is not secure, but confidentiality is assured.

Chapter Three

Outrageous Women

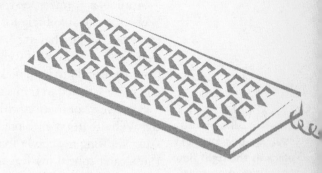

Y ou probably know at least a couple of people who have their own Web pages. Personal Web pages are like billboards on the information superhighway, in which individuals share writing, art, resumes, and autobiographical details with friends and strangers from around the world. At their best, these pages deliver insights, self-reflection, and social commentary on the level of a good print zine or an argument with a witty friend. At their worst, they ramble on in a self-indulgent fashion and make questionable use of precious bandwidth—do we really need to see so many photos of Fluffy the cat? In this chapter, we'll look at some of the sex activists, performers, and unsung exhibitionists who are taking their show onto the Web—informing, entertaining, and setting an outrageous example for the rest of us.

Star Personalities

If you're a woman author, artist, or activist whose beat is sex and sexuality, you learn to expect that your work will be regarded with equal parts ridicule and fascination. Whether your writing is trimmed by skittish editors, your funding withdrawn by irate politicians, or your courses protested at school board meetings, you get used to the fact that it's extremely difficult to get your message across in an unabridged form. No wonder, then, that female sex pioneers were among the first to start publishing on the Web—it offers an uncensored bully pulpit, an unlimited audience, and an unbeatable opportunity for self-promotion.

Among the articulate feminist pioneers putting up their own sex-related Web sites are authors Susie Bright and Nancy Friday, adult filmmaker Candida Royalle, and sex guru Annie Sprinkle. Along with other feminist writers and educators, they demonstrate by both word and example that, as Susie puts it, "Democratic access for women is revolutionary. Women have got to get in there and not hold back!"

Annie—a former porn star/prostitute turned artist/educator—sees the Web as an ideal vehicle for her philosophy of spiritual and sexual enlightenment: "I like that it's called the Web because the word *tantra* means web—you're weaving a web of energy on the web of the universe. I have a feminist agenda to help make the world a little bit freer, safer, more mature, and more satisfied in terms of sex."

After years of touring with her Post-Porn Modernist show, Annie "started the Web site in order to put my cervix on the Web as a conceptual art piece. After showing my cervix live to fifty thousand people in theaters, I thought: I just can't spread my legs anymore, but I still want to get my sex-positive message out there." With her site's "Public Cervix Announcement," Annie not only reaches women who have never made it to her shows but also places herself squarely in front of a global audience—an exquisite thrill for any performer. "There's something wonderful about knowing you're reaching a lot of people, even if you're just touching them a little bit," she explains. "As a prostitute I worked one-on-one. I had sex with three thousand guys, and I think I really touched them, in many cases in a meaningful way. But I'm not satisfied with only three thousand. I want to touch millions. Even if it's only a little teeny bit."

If Annie is using her site to reach out and touch millions of people at once, Susie Bright and Candida Royalle are using theirs to connect with individual readers on a more personal level. Susie's most popular page, "Why Me?" is a "rant about sex in America," which exposes common myths about sexuality (sex leads to irresponsible behavior, dirty movies lead to violence) and incites readers to write in with their own point of view. Susie comments that the feedback is particularly gratifying, because "You feel like you are finally meeting the people who actually treasure your work. It's so different from a bookseller's or reviewer's reaction. It's the real McCoy." And she encourages women seeking sex information online to take advantage of the interactive possibilities of the Web: "Don't hesitate to write the creators of any site to tell them what you think of it—they are people just like you who are much more accessible than the regular media."

Candida Royalle, best known for producing the Femme line of adult films "from a woman's perspective," is particularly accessible on her site. She dispenses practical sex advice to women and men via the "Ask Candida" Q&A column, which she uses as a forum to reinforce the message behind all her films: that women should rejoice in their sexuality. "Once a young woman wrote in saying, 'My boyfriend can't keep his hands off me, and I'm really into it, but I'm a little concerned—is there such a thing as too much sex?' So I wrote her back saying, 'Come on! You should hear the heart-wrenching letters I get from women whose men have no interest in them anymore. You are fortunate. As long as you're enjoying yourself, what's the problem here?' And a couple of weeks later, I got a message from her boyfriend saying that he had recognized the situation in my column, and he was so appreciative of and grateful for my response!"

As Candida's correspondent illustrates, women's experience of sex is often filtered through a diffuse anxiety that we shouldn't be enjoying "too much" pleasure. We are encouraged to think in this way by many societal messages, from the traditional "nice girls don't think about sex" to the more subtly disapproving "Shouldn't today's woman be concerned with more pressing social issues than sex?" The anxiety such thinking generates can manifest in self-censoring of sexual feelings. Feminist sexperts are quite familiar with censorship in all its forms, and they're used to eliciting a certain amount of dismissive scorn both from the mainstream media and from their fellow feminists. Nancy Friday recounts a relevant anecdote on her Web site about how she was snubbed by *Ms.* magazine upon the release of her groundbreaking book on women's fantasies: "When I called a woman editor and asked if *Ms.* would be interested in excerpting a section of *My Secret Garden*, I was informed, '*Ms.* will decide what women's sexual fantasies are.' When they reviewed the book several months later, the opening sentence was, 'This woman is not a feminist. . . .'" Not surprisingly, these sexperts revel in the luxury of having their own uncensored turf in cyberspace. As Susie notes, "The freedom I feel is one of the very, very best aspects of having my site. I've certainly run into censorship on other sites, such as my interview on AOL, where I wasn't allowed to say the word *clitoris!*"

And the more access women have to uncensored information and opinions about sex, the better. When we asked Susie what opportunities she felt the Web offered women, she answered cheekily, "Total world domination. Oh, I think the sky's the limit. I wish every woman was connected." But, as Annie notes, opportunities are accompanied by responsibility: "I'm tickled pink that anyone in the world can look at my cervix. After all, Carol Doda got arrested just for showing her breasts. But we have to keep doing the work and pushing the envelope. Now that women have certain freedoms, we have to exercise them or they're going to get taken away—the Web is a good place to do that."

Our only request of these online pioneers would be that they exercise their freedom of sexual speech a little more often! Many of these women update their Web sites infrequently and could stand to model themselves on the professional and amateur sex performers we'll discuss next, who are communicating almost daily with their online fans.

Professional Stars

Writers and artists aren't the only sex-positive women putting up their own Web sites. Some notable sex workers are also taking advantage of the Web's unique combination of safety and intimacy to build fan clubs online. The vast majority of female strippers, sex workers, and porn stars who appear on X-rated Web sites have nothing to do with the sites—as porn star Asia Carrera notes, "many of the girls who have Web sites have never actually been online." However, smart performers in control of their careers—such as Asia, stripper Danielle, bondage expert Lorelei, and the techno-savvy Danni Ashe and Madeleine Altmann—have figured out that maintaining a personal presence on their own sites inspires a loyal fan base that money can't buy. And it's a lot of fun.

As you might guess, the fans surfing these sites are the same ones patronizing female sex workers—that is to say, primarily straight men. But when men visit sites written and maintained by women, they receive as valuable an education as women visiting Nancy Friday's site—both men and women appreciate authentic (rather than scripted) expressions of women's sexuality. Men are eager to get a range of genuine perspectives on that ever-compelling question, "What do women want?" As one of our male survey respondents points out, "Women's viewpoints aren't represented enough. I'd like to know more about women, sex, and what really turns them on without male sexual fantasies interfering."

And women have a lot to learn from sex workers' sites, which provide a fascinating and demystifying look at the realities of the adult industry. Whether you're reading Asia Carrera's scathing comments on incompetent porn producers, Lorelei's behind-the-scenes account of filming a bondage video, or Danni Ashe's description of the Florida arrest that led her to give up a feature dancing career, you're getting a far more honest, well-rounded appraisal of sex work than you're ever going to find on TV or in the newspaper. And, through revelations such as Nina Hartley's description of her family's response to her career, you gain a better understanding of the

If we had a buck for every time a site's web-mistress or -master assured us that additions, upgrades, expansions, new interactive features, and corrections were just around the corner, we'd be rich women indeed. As surfing virgins we were oh-so-hopeful and naive, innocently trusting those seductive words—"live chat by next month," "major site redesign under construction," "hundreds of new links by spring"—but after months of repeat visits that yielded little or no change, we became hardened cynics. The truth is that the information superhighway is more like a truck-stop honky-tonk in a country-western song: littered with good intentions, broken promises, and unfulfilled dreams.

Time marches on offline but slows to a crawl on the Web, where six months can pass between issues of your favorite monthly e-zine. An online advice columnist's answer to your question about sex during pregnancy won't do you much good if it doesn't arrive until after your baby does. And countless anticensorship sites devoted to documenting the ongoing battle for freedom of expression haven't documented a thing since 1997, as if all clocks—and all threats to free speech—had stopped once the CDA was overturned.

So many sites are maintained as labors of love that it's no wonder well-intentioned hobbyists can't always keep their resolutions. We aren't blaming anyone whose site upgrades naturally take a backseat to priorities like holding down a job, raising kids, and enjoying a little offline recreation. But we'd prefer not to have grandiose plans dangled before us so temptingly. Promised improvements may hook a site one or two repeat visits, but if there's no follow-through, you'll alienate more readers than if you'd just waited to plug your new message board until after it was up and running. So use the time you spend posting those promises to get to work on the site!

women doing the work: "I don't throw what I do in the face of my family; they rarely see me in my full 'battle gear,' but I don't hide it from them either. They know about my three-way relationship, my swinging, my dancing, my talk shows, my movies and my college lectures. With the exception of my two brothers, I'd say my relationship with my family, including my grandmother until the time of her death at ninety-three, is excellent."

Amateurs: Everybody's a Star

Amateur sex sites are a true Web phenomenon. In the porn industry, "amateur" videos are low-budget productions staring nonprofessionals—they're basically X-rated home movies that mainstream adult companies distribute to an audience that values authenticity over gloss. On the Web, however, you don't need a distributor to reach an adoring audience; you just need an exhibitionist streak and a passing familiarity with technology. As a result, countless amateur sites, filled with explicit photos of women and men posed alone or in action with others, have flourished online. Many of these women first discovered the pleasures of displaying their assets to strangers by posting nude photos to Usenet newsgroups. Those who became well known and popular moved onto the Web.

Just as with professional sites, some amateur sites are simply photo galleries of a stable full of models and lack any semblance of personal touch. However, many are lovingly maintained by individuals who develop a genuine rapport with their fans. Some amateur sites are completely free, and some charge for members-only subscription areas to help cover maintenance costs.

Voyeurs who desire a truly up-close-and-personal look at their dream dates will appreciate the latest trend in amateur sites: webcams. On a webcam site, a video camera is hooked up to transmit regularly updated images of whatever is going on in front of the site owner's computer. These cameras don't operate with the speed of live streaming video (they refresh about once a minute), but they deliver a steady flow of photos of the site owner ostensibly going about an unedited life on screen. You may have heard of the more famous quasi-performance-art sites such as Jennicam or Kimiko-dreams—these have inspired a huge number of visitors who are just as likely to tune in on Jenni or Kimiko sleeping as sleeping around. Amateur exhibitionists are inclined to use their webcams more selectively and spicily for bedroom or shower scenes.

So, who are the women behind these amateur sites? They're the same women you see in line at the supermarket, pushing kids on the swings down at the playground, or talking business on their cell phones. They're just plain folks. Some enjoy the swinging lifestyle and sponsor contests in which fans win a chance to appear with them in the site's photos and videos. Veteran online exhibitionist Carol Cox helpfully includes photos of herself dressed in streetwear to help fans recognize her in public! Others are completely candid about their sexual unavailability, such as Maryland couple Jen and Dave, whose FAQ section includes this politely worded caveat: "The purpose of our page has always been the expression of Jen's exhibitionism, not swinging or meeting anyone in the 'real world.' We always hope that no one gets offended by this. It's just that we are essentially very private people. That's the beauty of the Internet."

What's particularly interesting about these sites is the level of intimacy that amateurs cultivate with their fans. These women don't feel compelled to compartmentalize their sexuality, separating it from the rest of their lives; some include details about their children, their pregnancies, and their professional projects right alongside their sexual fantasies. Think of how rare it is in our society to get such a range of information about another person, and how empowering it must be as a woman to present yourself in such a holistic way.

Again, women's amateur sites cater to a largely male audience, but we think they have something to offer other women as well. Visit a couple of these sites and think about how you'd choose to present yourself if you had your own Web page: What would you put in a FAQ section about your sexual interests and fantasies? What kind of photos would it turn you on to pose for? We're not suggesting that you're going to be so inspired by these sites that you'll want to whip out a webcam and start broadcasting explicit images of yourself to the world (though if you are, check out The Nose's HomeCAMs Page, p. 75, for technical tips). But at the very least you might begin to identify some of the ways in which you'd like to express your sexuality more openly. And maybe, just maybe, if you do have a Web page of your own, you'll be inspired to add a word or two about your favorite sex toy or that porn movie you watched over the weekend, right next to the photos of Fluffy. You'd be exercising the freedom that the Web provides, which would make us—and Annie Sprinkle—so proud!

Behind the Scenes with Danni's Hard Drive and Babes4U

We can picture the puzzled look on your face—you're wondering why you should be interested in sites with names like Danni's Hard Drive or Babes4U. You probably expect these sites to feature busty babes spouting inane dialogue ("please don't insert your floppy disk into my hard drive") and soliciting your money. What you probably don't expect is that these highly successful companies are both run by intelligent, savvy, sexy businesswomen.

Danni Ashe owns, stars in, and writes the code for Danni's Hard Drive, a predominantly soft-core site dishing up nude photos of delectable female models, chat, and live streaming video—a technology in which videos of explicit sex acts are transmitted live through the computer, and viewers can interact with the performers by typing in comments and requests. Madeleine Altmann co-owns Babes4U, a live streaming peep show featuring hard-core performances by a diverse cast of what Altmann affectionately refers to as her "babes."

Sure, these women operate mainstream adult sites that charge subscription fees, and yes, most of their patrons are men. But we think you should know about Danni and Madeleine because businesses like theirs are gradually changing the face of adult entertainment, for performers and consumers alike. Both women belong to a new breed of sex workers who are seizing the reins from men and starting up their own sites to the tune of "sisters are doing it for themselves." Strippers, nude models, phone sex workers, and porn actresses are flocking to the Web in search of better working conditions, greater exposure, and financial independence. With so many of these women succeeding on all three counts, one day you may see porn begin to reflect a more diverse and realistic portrayal of men's and women's sexual desires.

In the Beginning

A former erotic dancer, big-breasted model, and star of soft-core videos, Danni Ashe gave up the strip-club circuit after one too many grueling road trips and arguments with sleazy club managers. Bent on learning a new skill, she taught herself HTML (the Web's programming language) and moved her fan club online. The site's instant popularity—fueled initially by Danni's many fans on Usenet newsgroups, who spread the word about her site—convinced Danni that the Web was a superior way for erotic performers to pursue their trade, so she expanded her site to include photos and biographies of several dozen other models. Now she marvels that "online I can compete on the same level as *Playboy*, something that could never happen in the print world." Her instincts and hard work have paid off—Danni's site garners far more media attention than any online men's magazine, and she now hosts "*Playboy's* Hard Drive," a cable show about the most provocative sites on the Web.

No doubt Madeleine Altmann's masters degrees in interactive computer technology and video art propelled her into a career that would combine cutting-edge technology with her own exhibitionist tendencies. A shrewd businesswoman with a penchant for off-color puns and double entendres, Madeleine explains that after working as a porn model it became apparent to her that "If anyone should be profiting from selling female sexuality, it should be women." Since she "saw enormous growth (not just penile) and profit potential in the live streaming video market," she and partner Steffani Martin set up Madeleine's online show in 1996 with one hundred thousand dollars of their own money.

A Woman's Touch

Both entrepreneurs strive to create a style that distinguishes their sites from typical male-produced ventures. Danni's site is more visually distinctive— she offers tasteful, often playful, photos and biographies, a markedly feminine graphic style (pink and pretty), and some magazine-style content. Since Madeleine limits her services to live streaming videos of explicit sexual activity, her site has a more generic, let's-get-down-to-business look. What isn't necessarily visible to the outside observer is that both women are committed to giving their models and performers control over their work.

Danni's models retain complete control of their online image—they write their own biographies and choose which photos to present. As a result, you won't find the typical "I'm so horny for you, Daddy" tripe typical of many adult pay sites. Instead, viewers get a much more authentic and interesting peek into the lives and dreams of real women. Danni herself particularly enjoys the models' audio interviews (available in the members-only section), which she compares to "sitting quietly and listening to the grown-ups talk" when she was a girl.

Madeleine encourages freedom of theatrical expression, which, she's discovered, results in happy employees as well as satisfied customers. She explains, "We encourage the girls to get as wild as they want, which respects their individuality and gives them control, something men who are selling pussy sometimes forget to do. We give them lots of costumes with props and toys and wind up with some pretty kinky scenarios, which the customers love."

For the Boys

You won't hear any complaints from male subscribers. Sick of being stereotyped as stupid, undiscriminating, and helplessly horny by so many adult businesses, plenty of men patronize sites like Danni's Hard Drive and Babes4U because of the implicit respect they offer the viewer. "Men have been misjudged," says Danni. "They're not really looking for a cheap one-sided nude picture; they're much more interested in a three-dimensional fantasy." She goes on to explain that her site's most popular feature is the biographies—not the photos—of models, and that the most common request she receives is for more photos of models with their clothes on: "I have a theory about what happens when a man meets a woman. In the back of his mind he's wondering what she looks like without her clothes on, but once you show him a picture of the woman nude, then all he can think about is who she is and what motivates her to be naked for him."

After years of tapping into the complexities of the male libido, these women are ready to dispel some common misconceptions about male sexuality. "I think men are no longer threatened by intelligent, aggressive women either in front of or behind the camera," says Madeleine. "We choose models of all sizes, and we appreciate imagination as much as breast size. The customers really enjoy interacting with funny and smart babes." Perhaps this redefinition of what men want will ultimately improve women's sexual self-esteem by setting a more realistic standard of beauty and desirability. As Danni notes in her FAQ section, "I think any business can demean or exploit you if you let it. I personally feel fashion modeling is the most destructive thing to ever happen to women. It makes us all feel like we're inadequate because we're not six foot and one hundred pounds. In contrast, if you look at 'adult' modeling, there are hundreds of different publications glorifying the female form in all its different shapes, sizes, and colors."

Media Darlings

Men aren't the only ones getting turned on by Danni and Madeleine—the media is enjoying a love affair with them as well. From network news to talk shows to business magazines, the press can't resist the hook of a woman-run sex business, or as Madeleine explains dryly, "It's a perfect subject for the media because by profiling women in charge of their own sexuality, they can still use sex to sell a story without seeming exploitative." If anything, Danni and Madeleine are the ones exploiting the publicity machine in order to attract new customers and stay competitive in an overpopulated industry. Says Madeleine, "I'm much more of a media whore than I ever was an online slut."

Seducing the media isn't hard when you're a woman raking in big bucks selling sex to men through a medium that has been distinctly inhospitable to most commercial ventures. Most businesses that aren't sex-related have yet to eke out a profit from their Web sites, while Danni and Madeleine can't empty their pocketbooks fast enough. Although Madeleine won't disclose her income, she describes it as "quite substantial." Over the course of three years, Danni has watched her business snowball from a one-woman one-hundred-thousand-a-year start-up to a thirteen-woman, 2.7-million-dollar-a-year enterprise.

For the Girls

Although Danni and Madeleine have proven that women can be quite successful on the business end of adult entertainment, neither of them think that women are a potential market for pay sites such as theirs. Danni turned down an offer from Chippendales to create a site targeting women, because she just wasn't convinced there'd be a demand for it. She says, "I'd be clueless about how to do it, because I wouldn't patronize it. I'm interested, but not enough to pay." Maybe Danni senses the hesitancy of some women, such as one pragmatic survey respondent who said she wouldn't want to sign up for a pay site because "I'd feel I had to visit often to get my money's worth, and who wants to feel that eroticism is a chore?"

Madeleine offers her own colorful theory about why women wouldn't subscribe to pay sites: "I doubt there will be a big market for straight women wanting to see men, since for the most part they can do that for free. Ninety percent of the time if a women wants sex and goes up to a guy at a bar and says 'fuck me' she'll probably score, whereas a guy going up to a woman at a bar and saying 'please fuck me' will get a kick in the balls rather than a good balling." Whether these practical realities will keep women from paying for sexual entertainment online remains to be seen. Either way, both Danni and Madeleine believe the Web provides a tremendous opportunity for women to explore their sexuality and build their self-confidence in the process.

Role Models

Role models are in short supply, not just for female sex workers but for aspiring businesswomen and female techies as well. Danni is especially motivated to foster self-esteem and help other women forge successful careers in the adult industry. "As a nude model you're always getting the message that your life is worthless until you get out of the business," she explains. "I like what I do and am enjoying a fulfilling career—so I try to show the girls they can make something out of this work. I know girls who've gone on to create video companies and become agents and start Web sites. I use my Web site to help promote whatever it is the girls choose to go out and do."

In addition to promoting her models' professional endeavors on her Web site, Danni boosts their self-esteem in other creative ways. She invented the Sharon Mitchell National Human Services Award as a way of recognizing the achievements of sex workers who make contributions to their community (porn star Sharon Mitchell counsels drug-addicted youth). Danni sets a fine example of community service herself—in 1997 she organized a huge fund-raiser for an LA shelter for homeless teens. Sadly, the police threatened to shut down what was to be a nonexplicit performance, and the event was canceled, but not before Danni raised a substantial sum of money for the cause. Danni is also part of an ongoing dialogue with other online adult businesses interested in developing standards for responsibly presenting sex on the Internet.

If you're looking for role models who can talk the talk and walk the walk when it comes to sex work, neither Danni nor Madeleine will disappoint—they get right up on that virtual tabletop along with their employees. Erotic photos and videos starring Danni could keep you busy for weeks. Madeleine's sheer exuberance about crafting an erotic performance ought to inspire the exhibitionist in all of us: "I get a private booth with all these great toys so I really can get off . . . plus there are all these customers telling me how sexy I am. I really enjoy the creative element—not just the fantasies but the way I direct myself on screen." (If you're now rushing to your computer to subscribe to Babes4U, we should warn you that Madeleine's currently on a performance hiatus in order to devote more time to her new baby.)

When it's time to switch gears from erotic banter to technological jargon, these women talk shop about bandwidth, servers, and protocols like the pros they are. To retain maximum control over their sites, both women do their own programming, and they need to be ever-attentive to the latest technological developments in order to remain competitive. "The hardest part is when there is a 'spurt' of development in streaming technology and you have to scramble to upgrade your own system," says Madeleine, whose site is considered to be one of the most technologically sophisticated in the adult business. Madeleine has also developed and marketed software for companies that aren't sex-related.

You may or may not view Danni or Madeleine as role models, but you certainly can't argue with their job satisfaction. Danni says, "My favorite part of my job is being in control. I'm the master of my own destiny." And what works for her can work for others. Both of these remarkable women prove that there is a place for women online, whether they're in front of the camera, behind the scenes, or kicking back in front of a computer screen just enjoying the show.

A Word About Pay Sites

By now you may be intrigued by the prospect of viewing nude photos of your favorite celebrities, interacting with live erotic performers, or downloading pictures of an up-and-coming porn star. You can do all this and more—for a price. Adult entertainment sites offer such services in exchange for a subscription fee or pay-per-minutes charges—and subscribers are fueling a multimillion-dollar-a-year industry. But there's a downside. In the quest to make money, some companies are engaging in unethical business practices and have developed a new breed of technological trickery that will leave you cursing the day you laid eyes on a keyboard.

Most of these technological gimmicks are designed to transport you from the site you chose to another site. Why? Because the site you originally visited makes money each time you "click through" to the site of one of its advertisers. Click-throughs in the form of banner advertisements are employed by pay sites and free sites alike; you're probably familiar with these if you read any online publications—ads are one of the few ways in which free sites can generate revenues. However, certain less ethical adult sites use banner ads in a particularly deceptive way: in some cases, a banner ad that takes you to a new site is disguised as part of the original site, and you won't even know where you've ended up because the site locator name at the bottom of your frame won't show the new URL. You can get taken on quite a ride as you click around trying to get back to where you started, and needless to say, the original webmaster is making money off each click of your mouse.

Consoles—advertising windows that pop up on your screen whenever you enter or exit a Web page—are another annoying innovation: if you click on a console, it will either take you to a new site or sometimes link you back to the site you were trying to exit! These types of tricks can send you spinning in a loop (or "circle jerk") in which new frames blossom on your screen with every mouse-click, and you may well feel there's no way out. Often your only recourse at this point—if your computer hasn't already crashed under the onslaught of all the consoles—is to exit and then relaunch your browser.

A similar kind of circle-jerk involves "Top 50" lists. We can assure you that any adult site's claim to be a "Top 50" or "Top 100" site is a dubious distinction. Sites achieve their rankings on these lists based on the number of click-throughs they generate, a number that has nothing to do with quality and everything to do with how widely and deceptively they're advertised. In fact, many "Top 50" or "Top 100" sites earn their hits with completely fraudulent and tasteless come-ons, claiming to offer images of illegal sex acts (bestiality, incest, rape), celebrities, or—you guessed it—celebrities engaged in illegal sex acts!

The number of adult sites has surged since the Communications Decency Act was ruled unconstitutional; thousands of cheesy pay sites went up in 1997. There are an estimated twenty to thirty thousand adult sites as of this writing, but by this time next year many of these sites will either go under or be consolidated under a few owners. As Babes4U founder Madeleine Altmann comments, "The gold rush is somewhat over." The abundance of adult sites, the overload of sleazy click-through tricks, and an increasingly savvy customer base is probably going to burst the bubble for techno-scammers. With luck, the playing field will be left to those businesses that offer original content at a fair price.

Of course, we don't want to dissuade you from exploring every facet of erotic entertainment on the Web. To find legitimate adult sites, you can look for those that get high marks from independent reviewers such as Jane's Net Sex Guide (see p. 192) or that belong to organizations subscribing to certain basic business ethics such as the YNOT Network (see p. 78). And you can take the basic consumer precautions we're about to describe. If you're convinced you'd never pay for adult entertainment and are tempted to turn a blind eye to this section, you may want to think twice—the adult industry is pioneering commercial activities on the Web, and the same gimmicks employed by adult pay sites today may be employed by your favorite online magazine tomorrow.

Savvy Subscriber Tips
Before you sign up, we advise you to do the following:

• Find contact information. If there's no e-mail address or phone number, don't bother subscribing. If you have any questions about what you'll be getting and the terms of your contract, submit them via e-mail. The answer you receive, as well as the length of time it takes someone to respond to you, should give you a good idea of the company's commitment to customer service.

• Read the fine print. Make sure you understand the terms of your subscription agreement: the length of your membership, how you can unsubscribe, what the company is obligated to provide, and so on. As Jane from Jane's Net Sex Guide discovered, some sites promise the moon in their advertising but deliver substantially less: "The standard Terms and Conditions agreement we've found on adult Web sites specifically states that they do not have to provide the content they claim to provide in their preview!"

• Research the company's confidentiality policy. If you don't want your name and e-mail address sold to another company, make sure the site in question will honor this request.

• Beware of add-ons. You may be seduced by a site's low monthly fee only to discover that once you're a member you must pay extra for live streaming video, chat room visits, or other features. If it's not clear what your membership covers, ask in writing before subscribing, and save the written reply.

• Know the terms of the cancellation policy. Once you give your credit card to a pay site, most companies will renew your membership automatically each month, but they many require thirty days' notice to cancel. Similarly, if you're being offered a week's free membership, check the terms of cancellation—if you need to give seven days' notice, the week's membership isn't free! "The worst companies we found actually said in their terms that the first time you attempt to cancel, they may, at their discretion, upgrade your membership instead!" says Jane. "So, instead of canceling your bill, they'll actually bill you more."

• Be suspicious of outlandish claims. If it sounds too good to be true, it probably is.

If You Get Ripped Off . . .

If you feel you have been cheated, be a squeaky wheel. Start by e-mailing or calling the company and explaining your problem. If you get no response, threaten to file a complaint with your credit card company and the Better Business Bureau or the Federal Trade Commission (FTC). If that doesn't work, take the following steps:

• Complain to your credit card company. Write down your grievances and any action you've taken; send a copy of this documentation to your credit card company and a copy by registered mail to the offending site. Once the company knows that you've disputed the charges and that they'll be receiving a chargeback from the bank, they may finally respond. Rest assured that any credit card company has dealt with these situations numerous times and has no more interest in your subscription to the Sex Kittens site than in your subscription to *Scientific American*.

• Complain to the authorities. You can file a complaint with the attorney general in your state (Jane's Net Sex Guide provides links to attorney generals in all fifty states), or with the FTC. Don't let the fact that you were looking at naughty pictures deter you from standing up for your rights. Until enough people complain about shoddy business practices, adult companies won't have any incentive to change.

• Spread the word. Let others know about your experience. Many consumer sites, including Jane's, will post information about scams and bogus sites online.

• Know your rights. Visit one of the consumer resource sites listed on pages 77–78 to find out what other recourse you have.

Reviews

STAR PERSONALITIES

Anne and Cathy's Home Page

http://www.anneandcathy.com

Did you think we could write an entire book about sex on the Web without describing our own site? No way! We've written and edited three books together that have enhanced the sex lives of thousands of women and men around the world, but while other sexperts bask in the celebrity spotlight, we have toiled in relative obscurity. Until now! As you've probably gathered, our mission is to get the word out that SEX IS FUN, so our site offers sex-positive information, encouraging advice, opinionated rants, and ongoing site recommendations, in addition to rotating excerpts from our other books. Learn more about us—where you can find us online and off, what projects we're working on, and what sex toys we keep under our beds. Check out our photo gallery for proof positive that we really are two wholesome girls with friends, families, pets, and hobbies. We invite you to bookmark our page and let us continue to be your guides through the wide world of sex information and entertainment.

Gloria Brame's Castle in the Sky

http://gloria-brame.com

Poet and author Gloria Glickstein Brame's Castle in the Sky is, as she notes, an "eclectic literary site for free-thinkers." Enter the Castle and you'll find a wealth of pages reflecting her "frighteningly diverse" interests: contemporary poetry, technology, and the wide world of sexual dominance and submission. Gloria has been involved in online and S/M communities since before either were hip or mainstream, and she brings humor, good sense, enthusiasm, and a wide-ranging intellect to all her endeavors.

Gloria's autobiographical musings are engaging and well written; we particularly enjoyed her essays "Sex—Qu'est-ce Que C'est?" and "How a Nice Jewish Girl Like Me Became an Unrepentant Pervert." One wing of the Castle is devoted to the book *Different Loving: The World of Sexual Dominance and Submission*, co-authored by Gloria (with her husband, Will Brame, and Jon Jacobs). You'll find interviews from the book; a regularly updated newsletter; a graphics gallery featuring erotic photos and art from numerous artists; written erotica; photos of the Brames at play; and the well-organized Kink Links, containing over fifteen hundred links to fetish and S/M sites. Research for Gloria's latest book, *Consenting Adults: A Commonsense Guide to Kinky Sex*, gets its own page, and her "Dominant Ideas" page includes essays and how-to articles from a femdom point of view, along with transcripts of Gloria's weekly live chat sessions about BDSM on the "Kinky Pleasures" segment of Thrive/AOL.

Susie Bright

http://www.susiebright.com

"My site has no gizmos and no special effects, nor is it particularly picture-oriented. I was of the opinion that people online would give their eyeteeth for some first-rate reading material," says author, editor, porn critic, and well-known sexpert Susie Bright. If you crave reading material that will stimulate your brain as well as your libido, stop by Susie's friendly site and feast on her banquet of provocative essays, revealing interviews, book excerpts, and candid photos of Susie with family and friends. How about an explicit recounting of Susie's wet dream starring Dan Quayle? A poignant homage to Jimi Hendrix? A discussion of race and sexual stereotypes, or a heated attack on so-called family values? Whether you raise your eyebrows, laugh out loud, or shout in disagreement at Susie's opinions, you're bound to appreciate her willingness to tackle taboo or politically incorrect subject matter with her signature wit and verve.

Susie also posts a bibliography, videography, and frequently updated national tour schedule, so you'll always know where to find her. We only wish the reading material on this site were updated more often, but if you'd like a more regular Susie fix, check out her biweekly column on sex and popular culture for *Salon*, the Internet magazine (see p. 47).

Nancy Friday

http://www.nancyfriday.com

The author of groundbreaking books about women's and men's sexual fantasies (*My Secret Garden, Forbidden Flowers, Men in Love, Women on Top*), Nancy Friday offers an informative, interactive, utterly professional site. She is a tireless inquisitor—she wants your opinion on everything from reclaimed virginity to penis size to lesbian chic—and she usually posts a couple of the best responses (we would love to see even more). You can explore your fellow surfers' opinions in greater detail on the site's many discussion boards; the board devoted to sex gets quite a lot of activity. Nancy regularly responds to readers' questions, and she seems to be an active, enthusiastic presence on the boards.

Excerpts from her books, photos from her life, and an author interview round out the site. The themes that dominate her published books—beauty, power, sex, and mother/daughter relationships—get ample attention here. Nancy is outspoken, candid, and particularly engaging in reminiscences about the early days of her publishing career, when she blazed a trail for both the feminist and the sexual revolutions.

Candida Royalle's Femme

http://www.royalle.com

Candida Royalle's name would top any list of women who have influenced sexual entertainment and politics over the past twenty years. A former porn star turned producer, Candida launched her Femme Productions line in 1984 with the goal of creating erotic films "from a woman's perspective." Her videos emphasize women's pleasure and sexual self-discovery, are widely recommended by sex therapists for their positive role modeling, and have proved once and for all that yes, Virginia, there's a women's and couples' market for explicit entertainment.

Candida's site, a subsection of the Adam & Eve site (the current distributor of Femme videos), is easy to navigate and clearly organized. While updates are rare, the greatest activity is in the "Ask Candida" forum, in which Candida gamely answers questions from her fans: everything from industry-specific questions to sex advisor standards such as "Am I a lesbian if I fantasize about women?" or "How can I control the timing of my ejaculation?" We're not convinced that Candida's expertise and savvy is put to its best use providing generic sex advice, and we'd like to see her Q&A focus on adult filmmaking, erotic aesthetics, and gossip! For example, we love the site's "Behind the Scenes" section, in which Candida dishes the dirt about what goes on on the set of her movies (who knew that Candida herself sings on the soundtrack to *Urban Heat?*).

Annie Sprinkle's Homepage

http://www.heck.com/annie/sprinkleshow.html

Welcome to Annie Sprinkle's "intervaginal superhighway," where you're invited to enjoy a rest stop at the "Public Cervix Announcement"—a real photo of Annie's cervix accompanied by instructions on performing a cervical self-exam. This is just one example of the magic, humor, and passion for sex that this self-described "prostitute/porn star turned sex guru/performance artist" brings to the Web. "Annie's Wise Words" page includes her one-of-a-kind "Yoni Massage Ritual" (a detailed guide to masturbating yourself or a girlfriend), "40 Reasons Whores Are My Heroes," "101 Uses for Sex," and "How to Have an Energy Orgasm." You'd be hard-pressed to find issues of spiritual sexuality addressed so completely or with such endearing sweetness anywhere else online or off. A smattering of Annie's art is reproduced, but only enough to tease you into buying some of her books and "tit prints," which are available for sale through secure online ordering. Annie's impressive resume of

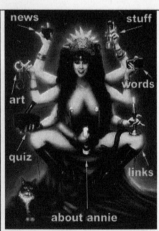

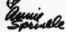

Welcome to the offical homepage of our favorite Prostitute / Porn Star turned Sex Guru / Performance artist ANNIE SPRINKLE.

This site offers background ABOUT Annie, her latest NEWS, an exhibition of her ART, a selection of her WORDS to the wise, plenty of LINKS to her favorite web sites, a QUIZ to determine your M.Q., and of course a huge selection of STUFF you can buy here online with our secured server or through the snail-mail.

For an automatic email catalog of Annie's stuff, email at: sprinkle@heck.com

Design: Katharine Gates, Gates of Heck Photography: Amy Ardrey Art Direction of Photo: Leslie Barany Over Painting: Ryszard Wojtynski film, video, and print appearances leaves no doubt about her vocation and should inspire you to heed her advice, such as "Learn About Your Breath: Sexual and orgasmic energy travel on the breath. Breathing techniques can make sex so much more powerful and satisfying. Rhythmic breathing is the best thing since the invention of the vibrator. It's possible to have an orgasm from breathing alone. Is this the safe sex of the future?"

Cecilia Tan's Homepage

http://www.circlet.com/pub/u/ctan/home.html

Writer, editor, and sexuality activist Cecilia Tan is the publisher behind Circlet Press, a small press devoted to erotic science fiction and fantasy. Her homepage, which is updated monthly, reflects her high energy and high output. It overflows with excerpts from her erotica and essays, "juicy personal details," journal entries, opinionated reviews and rants, and links related to interests from bisexuality and leathersex to Tae Kwon Do and wooden flutes. Fans will be pleased to check out Cecilia's schedule of readings and appearances and a bibliography of all her published work. You can also visit the Circlet Press site for information on ordering Cecilia's books, as well as publications from other small presses related to alternative sexualities (alas, online ordering is not yet a feature of this site).

PROFESSIONAL STARS

Danni's Hard Drive

http://www.danni.com

Sure, soft-core photos of beautiful buxom blondes are the engine driving this extraordinarily successful pay site, but owner Danni Ashe and her models deliver much more than the usual canned biographies and airbrushed close-ups. You'll find tasteful design, bountiful content in both the free and the members-only sections, and an overall approach that's best characterized as "girls just want to have fun." Danni posts regular interviews with her models and gives them free rein to write their own bios and select their own photos, so visitors to the site get to know something about the real women behind the cheesecake shots. Check out Danni's FAQ, which includes highly illuminating tips for guys (and gals) on "how to pick the perfect bra." A bloopers page adds humor, an online columnist facilitates discussions about sex-related news events, and Danni's well-archived press releases offer valuable insight

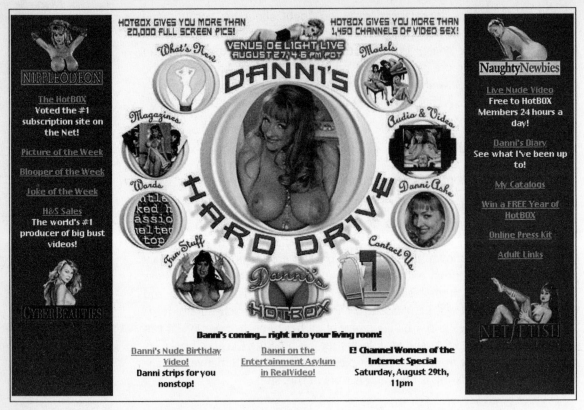

Copyright©Danni's Hard Drive—www.danni.com

into her mission, the sex industry at large, and the media's fascination with both. Subscribers gain access to live streaming video, a larger cache of photos, exclusive images from sex magazines, and audio interviews with the models.

Babes4U

http://www.babes4u.com

Owned and operated by two women, this live streaming video site has a slightly more sophisticated look than most adult pay sites—minimal banner ads, streamlined presentation, and performers who look like they enjoy their work. Visitors get very little free information—just a photo, a short biography, and a sample of dialogue from each of the site's main rooms, which offer the standard pay site options, including lesbians, hunky men (geared toward a gay audience), transsexuals, dominant women, and amateurs, all waiting to please. The performers are given artistic license, so Babes4U promises a spontaneous and creative online peep show.

Asia Carerra's XXX Buttkicking Homepage

http://www.asiacarrera.com

Meet the self-proclaimed "Nerd of Porn," Asia Carrera. Successful porn star by day and talented webmistress by night, Asia is the sole administrator and "cute dictator" of this entertaining site. Don't forget to review the rules of her "virtual aristocracy" before you enter: *do not* question her career choice; *do* agree to split the lottery money with her if you win. Once inside, you'll encounter a strong, opinionated, funny, smart, sexy woman, who is wildly successful at "stomping up and down on the stereotypical porn star bimbo image."

Asia's site offers a wonderful mix of porn trivia, self-revelation, and photos (from soft-core glamour stills to self-deprecating porno "Blooper Shots" to pictures of the star at home sans makeup). Check out her FAQ section and learn what porn stars get paid, what it's like to orgasm in front of the camera, and why she enjoys the business. Regular updates include a "Pic of the Week" and diarylike bulletins that run the gamut from news of her latest films to anecdotes about her personal life. Asia's site also includes a moderated chat room in which regulars (both men and women) discuss everything from the stock market to quantum physics to PMS. She helpfully includes her own rating system for the hundreds of videos she's appeared in, admits to her preference for couples flicks, and includes colorful notes about those videos she remembers best. Autographed Asia memorabilia—videos, CD-ROMs, photo stills, and lingerie—are available through secure online ordering, and a sex toy store is in the works. Aspiring webmistresses won't want to miss Asia's helpful programming tips.

Juliet's Boudoir

http://www.auntpeg.com

Juliet Carr is a veteran of what's known as the Golden Age of porn, which spanned the late '70s to the early '80s. She started her career at the age of forty and was best known for creating the popular character Aunt Peg, "a unique persona exemplifying the lusty, intelligent, self-assured older woman." She went on to produce and direct Nina Hartley's first video, *Educating Nina*, though disillusionment about how the video was edited caused her to leave the adult industry. In keeping with her trailblazing career, Juliet has since appeared in the independently produced video *Masturbation Memoirs* and has plans to revive her company, Afterglow Productions, in order to produce documentaries on sex and aging.

This site is infrequently updated, but we recommend you check it out if only to read "Porno Debut," in which Juliet tells the tale of how she shocked director Alex de Renzy by having an authentic orgasm during the filming of her first porn movie. You'll also find more recent gossip and anecdotes, as well as a small photo gallery, in which prints of Juliet are offered for sale.

Danielle's Fire

http://www.1dumblonde.com

The warning on Danielle's homepage notes, "This site may be considered offensive to some and/or detrimental to your conception of dumb blondes or bimbos." Indeed, this blonde, big-busted stripper will give your preconceptions a run for their money. Sure, she sells autographed photos and videos from the site, she features soft-core photos of herself messing around with her best friend, Brandy, and her diary consists largely of praise for and Polaroids of the big-name porn stars who have performed at the club where she works (the Pink Poodle in San Jose, California). *But*, you also get the "tip of the tongue" advice column, in which Danielle promises to answer all sex questions that aren't "too demented." Her advice is occasionally tongue-in-cheek, but she obviously takes the time to research many of the answers. (And our hearts go out to any sex educator who notes so politely, "Oh yeah, you guys who e-mail me pictures of your penises can stop!") We also loved Danielle's opinionated reviews of recent adult video releases, and her sex quiz, which we barely passed. (Did you know that in eighteenth-century Britain, "to make the chimney smoke" meant to give a woman an orgasm?) Don't feel bad if you score badly; Danielle dismisses high scorers with the comment "You are sooo cool! But you obviously don't have a life and have way too much free time on your hands."

Official Nina Hartley Home Page

http://www.nina.com/nina/index.html

If you believe the term *feminist porn star* is an oxymoron, you desperately need to pay a visit to adult superstar Nina Hartley's site. For over fifteen years, Nina has enjoyed a dual career as a polished, enthusiastic performer in adult videos and an articulate spokesperson for freedom of expression. Recently, she's branched out into directing and producing her own line of educational erotic videos (such as guides to anal sex, oral sex, and erotic dancing) for mail-order

While researching this book, we dutifully viewed a numbing array of mainstream adult sites, just to get the lay of the land. We found the predictable: "Oriental Love Doll" banner ads, the cyber-peep shows of live streaming video, and porn pay sites filled with generic publicity shots and star biographies lifted straight from press releases. And, to our huge relief and delight, we found the unpredictable: Asia Carrera's XXX Buttkicking Homepage.

Asia Carrera defies many porn star stereotypes. She's Asian (half Japanese, half German) in an industry dominated by the California blonde. She's ambitious and multitalented, and she's an unrepentant computer nerd. Most starlets whose names and images grace adult Web sites wouldn't recognize a computer mouse if it came up and bit them on the leg. Asia designed, programmed, and practically lives on her site—her personal touch has lured millions of visitors from around the world, and she enjoys the affections of a loyal band of online fans.

We asked Asia what inspired her to put up a site and received a typically breezy response: "I bought my computer for writing scripts. I was bored with that in two minutes and decided to figure out how to get online. Then I surfed around and decided that if every other weenie in America could make a site, so could I. At first, I just wanted to do it to say that I could, but then I got addicted, and now I can't stop."

Asia's site, which is updated weekly, is definitely addictive. She's intelligent, funny, impatient, unsentimental, and utterly revealing—about both her own personality quirks and the realities of life as a porn star. One of the most popular pages on her site is the "Bulletins" page, an online diary in which Asia divulges the details of her day-to-day life, from her dread of public appearances to her ex-husband's health problems to crises on the set of her latest flick to vacation plans with her boyfriend. And, as a visual counterpart, there are irresistible photos of Asia hanging around the house in jeans and combat boots, as well as blooper pictures from behind the scenes on porn sets.

Any visitor to Asia's site quickly learns that her interests include classical music (she's a trained pianist), physics, the stock market, and computers. She wears her perfectionist obsessions on her sleeve; she told us, "I hate when people e-mail me about spelling errors on my site, because I'm a spelling geek, and it's bad on the ego to know I put a typo out there for the world to see. I dash to fix the typo before I even finish reading the mail!" And she's dedicated to keeping her site free, though she has launched a hard-core archive entitled "Asia Carerra's Really Boring Pay Section" so that the "raincoat-wearing pervert can pay for my time slaving away on the free side."

Profile: Asia Carrera, Buttkicking Babe

Asia Carrera's XXX Buttkicking Homepage

http://www.asiacarrera.com

Profile: Asia
Carrera,
Buttkicking Babe,
continued

Noting that she prefers "living online to being in the real world," Asia spends a lot of time in her site's chat room. But, as pleased as she is by the devoted fans, business connections, and friends she's met and hangs out with online, Asia is most gratified by visitors who report that the tips on her "Webmaster" page helped them launch their own sites.

heavyweight Adam & Eve. Wondering how a former nurse and Berkeley-bred feminist became one of the country's most beloved porn stars? Read Nina's FAQ section to find out. One of the few out bisexuals in mainstream porn, Nina is open about her three-way marriage (to husband Dave and wife Bobby) and is both down-to-earth and encouraging about the swinger's lifestyle.

With the exception of a couple of photos of Nina's famous blue eyes and equally renowned heart-shaped butt, her simple, infrequently updated site is text-only. However, we consider it a must-see. The merely curious should check out Nina's FAQ section and copies of articles by and about her career at least once. Fans can sign up for her fan club and revisit the site for regular updates to her touring schedule and links to sites related to current projects.

Lorelei's Bedroom Bondage

http://www.bedroombondage.com

This heartwarmingly candid site, formerly known as Kristine Imboch's Bedroom Bondage, is devoted to one bondage aficionada's passion. Lorelei has been making bondage videos for over ten years, and she is a knowledgeable, friendly spokesperson for what is both her livelihood and her fetish. Along with the usual links, photos, chat, personals, and message board (much of the site is free, but members get access to premium photo layouts), Lorelei includes diary excerpts, an excellent FAQ section, and the "Dr. Bondage" column featuring her own safety tips. Smart and self-aware, Lorelei isn't afraid to examine what's behind her fetish, and diary entries such as the following make for intriguing, enlightening reading: "Like many women, I now find it's not easy to relax and open up to arousal. It's easier if a man takes control and coaxes me into giving my passion into his possession. Bondage allows me to play this role. It also helps me block out distraction and focus on sensation—mental abilities sometimes difficult in a non-bondage moment." Lorelei's new site, www.forcefantasies.com will feature romantic ravishment fantasies.

Carol Cox's Wild Rose

http://www.carolcox.com

A dedicated swinger out of Montreal and one of the first online exhibitionists.

Jen n Dave's Homepage

http://www.jen-dave.com

A cute twenty-something couple; all photos are of Jen.

Jenni

http://www.jennicam.org

The college student who launched a thousand webcams with her site.

Kimiko

http://www.kimiko-dreams.com

Guests get a free glimpse into Kimiko's life; members get live streaming video.

The Nose's HomeCAMs Page

http://www.homecams.com

Several hundred listings of webcam sites and tips on how to create your own webcam, including detailed hardware reviews.

Oasis

http://mirage.skygate.net

An extremely popular amateur, Oasis tours the country regularly to add new material (and fans) to her site.

Bernadette Taylor: The Diary of a Virtual Girlfriend

http://www.sitepool.com/bernadette

Bernadette discovered her vocation as an online exhibitionist when she began posting photos to Usenet newsgroups, and she's since moved her unique blend of good humor, high spirits, and fetching soft-core photos onto the Web. It's unusual for an amateur site with so many features to be completely free: you'll find photos, FAQs on all aspects of sexuality, erotic stories, chat, a webcam, games, and more. Bernadette is up-front about the fact that she's engaged, the mother of a toddler, and unavailable to her fans in RL (real life), but she takes her responsibilities as a virtual girlfriend quite seriously.

Scratch the surface of this charming Australian exhibitionist and you'll find a natural-born sex educator. Bernadette has carefully organized all her responses to fans' questions into specific FAQs (on genital shaving, anal sex, oral sex, and more) and suggests that you "try reading them with a partner and use them as a forum for discussion." And she manages to work some gentle instruction into all the personal questions she receives, for example, "Yes, I have an eight-month-old daughter. Being pregnant didn't affect my sex drive at all . . . and having a child hasn't either. Some mothers get tired and tend to lose their sex drive . . . before men complain, they should help out more with the kids so she isn't so tired."

Virtually Venus—Gorgeous Goddesses

http://www.vvenus.com

"On a remote island in the middle of the tumultuous Information Ocean there exists a secret clan of Sirens, Sybils and Cyber Goddesses whose only concern is the wanton pursuit of pleasure." The sexual and the spiritual meet headlong within the Temple of Love, an exceptional amateur site filled with original erotic photos of seven "playful and lusty divine creatures" romping with one another and with men friends. These beautiful, completely natural (no silicone, no big hair) women believe that sex is sacred, and their exhibitionism is downright intoxicating. While their online magazine is available to members only, plenty of free material is posted on the site: from an explicit slide show of hard-core images to their *Mindf*ck* e-zine, which includes a gallery of Venus art through the ages, excerpts from the metasexual writings of Marco Vassi, general philosophical ramblings, and links to related sites.

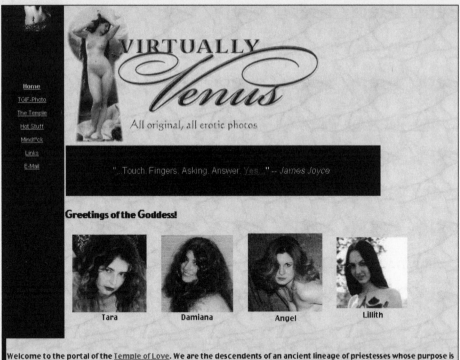

Copyright©Aisha Qadisha

CONSUMER RESOURCES

Better Business Bureau

http://www.bbb.org

Offers consumer tips and accepts complaints.

Consumer World

http://www.consumerworld.org

Provides links to a plethora of consumer information and organizations.

Federal Trade Commission

http://www.ftc.gov

Reports online scams, offers buying tips, and outlines mail-order regulations.

Internet Fraud Watch

http://www.fraud.org

Accepts reports of fraud and posts consumer alerts.

Jane's Net Sex Guide

http://www.janesguide.com

A great source of tips for adult consumers. Jane is proactive in researching and exposing online scams.

YNOT Adult Network

http://www.ynotnetwork.com

A network of adult sites following good business practices.

Chapter Four

Sex Information

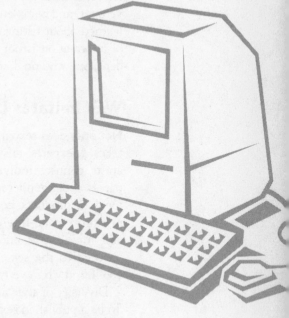

Since we began the twentieth century fleeing Victorian sexual repression, it seems only appropriate that we fly into the twenty-first on the wings of a technology that has the power to free us from sexual shame and ignorance. The World Wide Web offers unprecedented access to a plethora of sex information; the more we avail ourselves of this, the greater our chances for healthy and satisfying sex lives.

Information about sex abounds on the Web, covering just about every subject imaginable. Got a question about STDs? Looking for tips on creative foreplay? Researching a paper about sex laws around the country? Want to read some honest reviews before buying a good sex book? Finding these resources—and more—is not only possible on the Web, it's a whole lot easier than relying on traditional methods.

In the offline world, getting your sex questions answered requires persistence and nerve, assuming you know where to look and whom to ask. As sex therapist Al Cooper puts it, "If you're cooking and need a recipe, you can ask your mother, you can ask your next-door neighbor, you can ask somebody sitting next to you at work, but if you want to know something about sexuality, whom do you go to? You probably can't ask your mom, you're ashamed of asking your next-door neighbor, and you're reluctant to ask your physician."

That leaves you to dig for the answers yourself, often an equally unappealing option, as one survey respondent points out: "Given the amount of time it takes to locate anything useful in the library, I usually don't bother." As a result, many of us go without information that could improve our sexual health and our skill as lovers. The Web changes all that by offering free, convenient, and completely private access to important educational materials. "I learned about fisting, the G-spot, and female ejaculation online—that kind of information is not easy to find where I live," says another survey respondent, one who no doubt owes an orgasm or two to the Web.

Web Imitates Life

Not only does sexual content vary enormously online—so does the form it takes. "Sexperts" answer questions that Dear Abby *never* gets to field, therapists counsel individuals in online sessions, students post their thesis papers about gender and sexuality, sex boutiques detail ways to use and care for their products, condom makers report up-to-the-minute safer sex information, special-interest groups offer sex-positive resources and referrals—and for all you know, your next-door neighbor may have a Web site devoted to the secrets of satisfying sex. This variety virtually guarantees you'll find whatever you're looking for, plus a whole lot more.

Diversity of style and content sets the Web apart from traditional media. To be a published sex book author, you usually need a degree, credential, or area of expertise; but to be a Web site author, all you need is minimal start-up equipment and something to say. As a result, individuals with a range of sexual interests, attitudes, and levels of experience share their tips, opinions, and support with others online. Since many sites evolve out of the personal experiences of their creators, surfers get a direct line into the bedrooms—and the brains—of folks across the world. Janis Maria Cortese, one of the creators of Web by Women for Women, a site dealing with sexuality and censorship issues, describes the organic way the contributors to the site choose their material: "One of us will use a new product for her period, and that will spawn a topic. Recently, someone had some discomfort during sex, and we researched ways to make it more comfortable, and the vibrator page was born. We started chatting about losing our virginity and realized we all had unresolved issues that other women and girls probably had, so we added a page on that."

Read the paper, turn on the TV, or pick up a magazine, and there's a seemingly endless stream of sex surveys and statistics that define the parameters of "normal" sexual behavior. On the Web, you'll get an entirely different perspective on what sexual issues and activities are the norm for women and men around the country. While the predominance of "all-nude girls" sites catering to male fantasies may not surprise you, the hundreds of sites related to BDSM (erotic power exchange) suggests that practices you might consider "fringe" are, in fact, quite common. A volunteer at the Society for Human Sexuality, a site that boasts the largest collection of online texts devoted to sex, explains, "The volume of BDSM writings on our site is driven by our general interest in covering topics as completely as we can, the quantity of material that BDSM enthusiasts have produced, and the explosion of creativity and interest that has occurred around this particular community in the last several years." Or, as one of our survey respondents points out, "What mainstream society sees as abnormal is in fact normalized on the Internet."

Exposure to such a rich spectrum of sexual preferences can have unexpectedly pleasurable results. If you've always harbored a secret desire to be tied up, discovering like-minded people on the Web may be all it takes to inspire you to practice a little restraint in the bedroom. Before you know it, a whole new dimension of fantasy, role-playing, and sexual experimentation can open up for you. This comment is typical of the many survey responses we received describing a pattern of sexual discovery, exploration, and liberation: "Though I'm pretty vanilla in my tendencies, the stories and information I've read online have made me more experimental in my own sexuality than I ever thought of being on my own."

In addition to enhancing your own sex life, exposure to a variety of sexual tastes can also breed tolerance, understanding and acceptance of others, as this respondent clearly demonstrates: "I found some very good tips about fellatio and cunnilingus from the Web, which my wife and I practiced. Later I understood they were written by homosexuals and realized that they must be the real experts, having experience from both ends, so to speak. This has profoundly changed my attitude toward homosexuality in a positive way."

For sexual minorities, the Web offers hard-to-find information, a welcoming fellowship of peers, and a sense of safety that is not always available offline—which could explain why sites created by and for gay, lesbian, bisexual, and transgendered communities are among the most highly visible sex information resources online. As the editors of the e-zine *mouth organ* note, the ability to do grassroots publishing and organizing on the Web has made it a particularly potent resource for members of marginalized sexualities: "There are at least two areas we can think of where the bulk of sex information is online, no choice about it: polyamory and transgender issues. You could go crazy looking for print materials that specialize in either of these areas. BDSM is another area that's basically converted to Web-based sources in a big way. Our standard theory is, the more underground the practice is, the more Web information it'll have." The Web has been a particu-

WHAT WOMEN WANT

"I'd like to see an abundance of explicit photographs and a site that caters to a large variety of sexual expressions, not necessarily politically correct material. Most educational sites take themselves too seriously and don't include the hard-core sexy stuff. I think a site could offer both, and people would take more interest in the advice if they also saw how much satisfaction can be gotten out of it."

larly valuable tool for the transgender rights movement, connecting other-wise isolated individuals to a national network of information sharing, legal watchdogging, and political activism.

While gay, lesbian, and bisexual sites often focus primarily on lifestyle and political issues, we hunted down a few that celebrate the "sex" in "sex-ual preference." In her site, WOMB, Kelly Garland includes sex instruction tailored to lesbians, because "It brings me great joy to know I have in some small way helped another woman discover a new sexual aspect of herself." Whether you're on that path to self-discovery or you're merely curious about what lesbians do in bed, you'd be hard-pressed to find a more elo-quent description than this excerpt from Garland's site: "Lesbian sex is not as simple as a tongue sliding into a vagina. It is about strap-ons, about bending over with a smile on your face, about knowing she's going to bring you to the edge and back again. It's about knowing your needs—and hers—are going to be met. It's about recognizing those masculine and feminine qualities in her, qualities that we all embody but play out in different ways. It's about the recognition of fantasy and dark, dirty little turn-ons that we aren't supposed to articulate. It's about honesty, trust and love."

The Doctor Is Always In

"Different Web sites have taught me a ton about STDs—things I never learned from high school, college, television, advertisements, doctors, or any other resource," says one survey respondent. Access to accurate sex informa-tion allows each one of us to make informed decisions affecting our sexual health that, in many cases, can be the difference between life or death. Current information about birth control and safer-sex activities can prevent unwanted pregnancies and disease transmission, as well as assist those who are pregnant or infected to resume a safe and satisfying sex life. In addition, since anyone with Internet access can communicate easily with others around the world, individuals with common health concerns are now net-working like never before—swapping advice, encouragement, and practical resources. For groups whose sex lives have traditionally been ignored by the medical establishment, such as people with chronic disabilities or illnesses, this grassroots information sharing is uniquely life-enhancing.

And let's face it—in person, it's never easy to ask a doctor or health pro-fessional a question about sex. But it is online. You don't have to worry about blushing, mumbling, or chickening out—just type up your question and send it off anonymously to one of the many sex advice sites on the Web. Al Cooper, the sex therapist behind *Self-Help and Psychology's* Q&A column, claims that "questions submitted online tend to be much more explicit" than in his offline practice, even than those mailed to his print column for *Men's Health* magazine. The anonymity and immediacy of asking a question on the Web clearly relaxes people's inhibitions.

Replies are usually posted on the site for the edification of all viewers, along with archives and FAQ sections featuring past questions. Archived Q&A columns and sex FAQs contain a gold mine of information on every conceivable sex subject—you can use them to improve your general knowledge about sexuality as well as to seek answers to specific questions. There may seem to be a glut of advice columnists online, but you can take advantage of the situation to shop around for those whose tone and attitude suit you best. We provide excerpts from several different Q&A columns (p. 102) in order to demonstrate the variety in style and approach.

Unfortunately, the lag time between submitting your question to a sexpert and having it answered can be the online equivalent of waiting for a doctor's appointment or being put on hold indefinitely. We sent questions to half a dozen online columnists and only two—from Ask the Couch! and the Coalition for Positive Sexuality—responded within two weeks. Many advisors receive so many questions that they can't answer them all, so there's a good chance that yours will get tossed in the dead e-mail file. If the information you're looking for isn't already posted and you need it in a hurry, you're probably better off calling a sex information hotline or speaking to a health professional.

A Word of Caution

Critics of the Web often point out that the downside of democratic information sharing is that misleading or potentially harmful material can't easily be distinguished from fact. Because there are no standards, no tests, and no minimum credentials required, anyone can pass themselves off as an expert. We have yet to run across any instances of intentional deception, but be aware that you'll encounter your fair share of opinions that come off sounding like fact. Even then, in most cases, either these individuals clearly admit that they're stating an opinion or it's obvious from their writing style that they're standing on a soapbox, not sitting on a medical review board.

If you want to minimize the risk of getting bogus information, there are a few things you can do. Stick to sites that have an affiliation you recognize and trust. Universities, nonprofits, professional organizations, and reputable companies often provide links to other sites that have earned their endorsement. On unfamiliar sites, look for a mission statement or a note about the author's intentions or qualifications. But please don't dismiss a site simply because its author doesn't have a degree or professional credential. Many lay people (ourselves included) are perfectly capable of sharing excellent advice based solely on experience and perspective. However, if your question requires a medical opinion, you should probably stick to sites featuring licensed health professionals; those with unlicensed sexperts usually have a clearly stated policy of not dispensing medical advice. In either case, we strongly encourage people with medical problems to see a physician. Ultimately, as this survey respondent explains, common sense is your best defense: "I take a lot of the sex stuff with a grain of salt and trust my judgment about how 'real' some of the information is."

For the Love of Sex

As you surf the Web, you may wonder what motivates the individuals behind these sites to devote so much time and energy to endeavors that bring little, if any, financial gain. Most do the work out of a simple desire to further sexual discourse.

As members of the scientific community discovered decades ago, the Internet affords an incredible opportunity to collaborate with colleagues. In 1990, Carnegie Mellon posted a collection of humanities texts on its interactive Web site, The English Server, so that students and professors could research, critique, and correspond with one another about their work. Today the site is home to hundreds of engaging and provocative papers on a variety of subjects, including gender and sexuality.

Sex therapists and other health professionals are beginning to take advantage of the Internet's networking and educational capabilities. Judy Siefer, a sex therapist and co-founder of Sexhomepage, one of the most ambitious archives of sexuality references online, is part of a "virtual office" with staff in Florida, Utah, and West Virginia. She found herself drawn to the Internet after talking to a female client who enjoyed a satisfying sex life based entirely on writing and posting slash fiction online (*slash* is the term for a genre of erotic fiction that revolves around popular TV characters and often has a homoerotic theme): "I realized there's this whole world of sex out there I hadn't a clue about! And that's what hooked me. As a therapist, I figured I better find out what the hell was going on." Now she sings the praises of the Web's potential as "an interactive encyclopedia of sex information."

But the number of academics and professionals online pales in comparison to the countless number of individuals with passionate personal agendas who delight in using the Web as a sounding board. For example, Janis Maria Cortese, the author of the sexuality pages at Web by Women for Women, believes that providing women with a forum to discuss their sexuality is the best way to subvert the censorship that has traditionally confined women's sexuality. Explains Janis, "The right wing clucks its tongue and says, 'Oh, but the life of a woman is Such a Trial, so just Learn to Make Do.' The left wing *refuses* to confront the issues. Emotional and physical and spiritual issues surrounding sex for women involve a lot more than goddamned birth control pills, medical terminology, and specula. We've got more ubiquitous concerns about unfulfilling sex than just what falls under the heading of rape. Fulfilling, wonderful, life-improving sex is *not* merely that which is left when rape has been cut out of the picture!"

Kelly Garland's site, Womb, evolved out of her desire to put a more human face on the ever-expanding gay and lesbian online community. "My inspiration came from the fact that too many of the queer and/or lesbian sites out there were lacking in individuality," she says. "Far too many rainbows and not enough guts. When I surf, I like to think I'm seeing some aspect of that person's life—their aesthetics, ideologies, and opinions—not just emblems or the iconography of their community."

Of course, many folks talk about sex on their Web pages because it's just plain fun. Some even get class credit for it! The Society for Human Sexuality's Web site began as a student project at the University of Washington in 1995 and is now widely recognized as the best collection of sexuality materials online. "I see our Web site as an example of what can happen when 'what you like to do' coincides with 'what other people value,'" says one of the group's volunteers. "Time that would have been spent watching TV shows or mindlessly surfing the Web got redirected into writing and *purposefully* surfing the Web, not out of 'duty' but out of the sheer pleasure of creating and organizing information on a wonderful topic."

Sex *is* a wonderful topic, and you deserve to know as much about it as possible. The sites reviewed in this chapter encompass a tremendous variety of interests and meet our standards for accuracy, enthusiasm, and sheer inspiration, as do the informational sites and gateway resources you'll find in other chapters. Equipped with such an abundance of sex information, you're more than ready to enjoy the delicious sex that awaits you in the new millennium.

Reviews

SEX INFORMATION

American Sex Machines

http://www.levins.com/sexmachines.html

Wow the guests at your next dinner party with your impressive knowledge of sex machines. Whet their appetites with tales of self-stiffening condoms and coital couches, but leave the description of the contraption designed to cure wet dreams until after dessert. Just the thought of tweezers tugging at their pubic hair during nightly erections could kill your male friends' appetites. Hoag Levins, the author of *American Sex Machines: The Hidden History of Sex and the U.S. Patent Office,* presents several short excerpts from his book, plus illustrations of a dozen sex machines—you'll have to buy his book to read about the other eight hundred! The history of these patented sex toys reveals the evolution of sexual mores and practices from the 1840s to the present. Not surprisingly, sex-prevention devices dominate, but sex toy lovers will rejoice that the "massage tube with hand grip" caught on and is better known today as that perennial pleaser, the penis pump.

Crave

http://www.webmistress.org/crave

If you have questions about the appeal of submissive sexuality, visit the site of this charmingly candid lesbian submissive, who refers to herself here simply as "Crave." She has assembled a useful array of articles and essays defining and demystifying BDSM, accompanied by her own erotica, photos of lesbian S/M, a good set of annotated links, and quirky tidbits such as a list of recommended music to play during an S/M scene.

Dr. Eleanor Hamilton

http://www.ptreyeslight.com/columns/hamilton/hamilton.html

She may be in her eighties, but Dr. Hamilton is just as comfortable explaining transsexuality as she is discussing creative sex for the elderly. This sex therapist, marriage counselor, and author has earned her place in history as a pioneer of sexual liberation and a lifelong advocate of sex education; her "Loving and Living" columns from the *Pt. Reyes Light* weekly newspaper are reproduced here in their entirety. These columns, which cover issues related to sexuality, parenting, and relationships, overflow with the sage advice, gentle guidance, and welcome pragmatism that befit a sex scholar and grandmother. Who among us wouldn't have benefited from the straight sex advice dispensed in one of her columns, "Letter to My Granddaughter": "With his hands, he can caress your clitoris and vagina, bringing you to ecstatic orgasm. And the miracle is that you can delight in each other's bodies safely: no unwanted babies, no death dealing AIDS, no venereal disease. Even better, using this means of sexual togetherness, you both learn how to be more skillful lovers who can satisfy each other far more effectively than if you had just indulged in the 'put-it-in' variety of sexual activity."

Elf Sternberg's Alt.Sex FAQ

http://www.halcyon.com/elf/altsex

Before the alt.sex newsgroup became inundated with spam, legions of men and women whiled away their online hours conversing about technique, sharing resources, and exploring facets of their own and one another's sexuality. Several of the participants, including this site's archivist, Elf Sternberg, culled the best from those discussions and compiled the alt.sex FAQ. The result is a no-nonsense, nonjudgmental instruction manual that covers the vocabulary of sex, anatomy, sex toys, first-time sex, sexual positions, anal sex, oral sex, STDs, and safer sex (among other things!). The anatomy lesson is accompanied by real photos, including depictions of a circumcised and an uncircumcised penis. If high school sex education programs went beyond simple explanations of reproduction, this FAQ would be on the required reading list. The only thing the site lacks is a supplemental list of resources. Elsewhere on Elf's site you'll find the extensive "hanky code guide" as well as an abundance of erotic fiction (with a science fiction slant). This "historical document of the golden years" of alt.sex has not been updated since 1994, but most of the content is of timeless value.

English Server

http://eserver.org

Where else can you find a paper about female strippers from a pro-sex feminist point of view, an essay about fetishizing frat boys, an analysis of lesbian imagery in mainstream media, a girls' guide to condoms, and a hysterical discussion of homoeroticism in Batman films (called "Holy Homosexuality, Batman!"), all archived together? The English Server was created by humanities students at Carnegie Mellon who discovered the Internet provided an ideal forum for peer review and discussion of their materials. The result is an incredibly diverse body of scholarship, art, journals, and novels, with over eighteen thousand listings (yes, there is a search function!). The "Gender and Sexuality" section focuses on discussions of sex, gender, sexual identity, and sexuality in cultural practices. Visitors are invited to submit their own material to the collection and will find links to academic organizations, mailing lists, and conferences.

Heartless's Holey Haven

http://www.grownmencry.com/hhh/HHH.html

This "haven for holes and things that go in holes" offers an irreverent look at women and sex. You'll never experience a dull moment while browsing the Holey Haven, designed by a woman for women (and men who can take a good joke). You will have one belly-aching laugh at the "stupid penis tricks," which are submitted by readers and illustrated by the webmistress herself. These submissions prove you can teach an old dog new tricks—just try dressing your favorite member up as a troll or a puppy dog, or teaching it how to fly, dance, or disappear.

More serious students of sex will appreciate the essays "Hats off to Cocksuckers," "Muff Divers of the World," and "When a Blow Job Is Just a Job," which offer tips on giving great head—from using all your senses to enhance sex to gracefully removing pubic hair from between your teeth. Other essays and a Q&A section discuss technique, etiquette, and relationship concerns in the same spirit of fun and frankness. If you're looking to expand your sexual repertoire with some sizzling suggestions, "Smokin' A-Z" offers plenty of role-playing scenarios, while "Searchin' for Smoke" chronicles the webmistress's quest for porn. Let your imagination run wild in the "Penis for a Day" section—filled with photos of phalluses and the ramblings of women describing what they would do if they had one of their own. Stunning visual presentation, with lots of erotic, explicit photos of men and women, many of whom are engaged in some form of penetration.

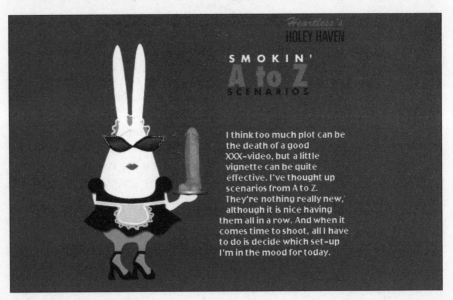

Copyright©Heartless's Holey Haven

Home Arts: Kissnet

http://homearts.com/depts/relat/00dprec1.htm

If you prefer your sex tips straight out of women's magazines, this is the site for you. The Hearst Corporation's Web site combines features from several of its magazines, devoting a special section (called "Kissnet") to love, sex, and marriage. *Redbook's* "Sex and Marriage" archives yield some valuable pearls of wisdom, such as tips on talking dirty and different styles of lovemaking. You'll also find a popular discussion forum and chat room, including one discussion board called "he said/she said," where men and women compare notes on sex. Expect lots of romance and dating advice, as well as—you guessed it—quizzes about compatibility!

"I haven't seen a web page yet that deals with the nitty gritty of giving him a blow job. I'm not talking techniques. Or whip cream usage. Or how to be a porn queen in three hours. I'm talking SURVIVAL SKILLS and SOLUTIONS. After all, you don't want him to take his toy and go home, you just want him to play nicer. . . "

For details on these fellatio survival skills (which cover gagging, swallowing, and dealing with stray pubic hairs), you'll have to pay a visit to Heartless's Holey Haven, which bills itself as a "haven for holes and the things that go in holes." If you need help translating, that means a site about female sexuality with an emphasis on penetration!

It's Heartless's highly personable blend of sex advice, entertainment, and humor that makes her site engaging as well as instructive. She offers great primers on oral sex, a moving tribute to foreplay, her own guide to sexy smut, and a nice dose of explicit imagery. "It's a desert out there, and we're thirsty," she says by way of explaining her site's popularity with women.

She chose the name Heartless to use on her site because "Mama raised me to be such a nice, polite girl, which can be a real handicap sometimes. With a name like Heartless, no one expects you to be nice, and I can discuss sex and my opinion of it without having to consider anyone else's feelings." It's her frankness and willingness to share her own desires and opinions that give her site such a bite, as well as refreshing authenticity. What porn-loving woman wouldn't appreciate her "Requirements for Smokin' Hot Videos," which include demands of equal time for oral sex, along with the eradication of high heels and long fingernails!

For sex humor that would make David Letterman blush, check out Heartless's collection of "Stupid Penis Tricks," with illustrations by the

Profile: Heartless Heartless's Holey Haven

http://www.grownmencry.com/hhh/HHH.html

Profile: Heartless
Heartless's Holey
Haven, continued

author. You'll find instructions on how to transform your favorite penis into Einstein, Frosty, or Godzilla, use it as a ring toss or a towel holder, or teach it to dance and serve candy. Heartless conceived of the idea one sleepless night as a way of helping her cope with negative feelings caused by past sexual abuse. "I knew for my emotional well-being I had to get a healthier perspective on hard-ons, because they were not all evil," she explains. "'Stupid Penis Tricks' began as therapy, helping me laugh and have fun in a loving way with Mr. Happy. It worked." It's resonating with others as well: "Stupid Penis Tricks" became such a hit that readers started sending in their own ideas, and magazines like *Playboy* and *Penthouse* have featured the little guys. Heartless illustrates all the ideas she posts and has started a business called Makes Grown Men Cry, which produces an annual calendar of the best penis tricks.

Whether she's dressing up a penis as a shrimp cocktail or doling out cunnilingus tips in "Muff Divers of the World," Heartless proves you can find both sexual empowerment and erotic inspiration on the Web. "Being able to combine my art and my words into one form has been an incredibly freeing experience," she says. "In a society where women tend not to have power, a personal homepage has given me confidence and a chance to meet wonderful women."

Jackin' World

http://www.jackinworld.com

Designed originally as an informational site for young boys with questions and concerns about masturbation, this site has skyrocketed in popularity and now claims a readership between the ages of eleven and eighty. An extensive index covers common concerns from acne to wet dreams, answering questions about guilt, technique, and penis size along the way, and the excellent illustrations of male genital anatomy are a valuable accompaniment. Active visitor participation includes numerous first-person accounts, as well as separate chat rooms for the under- and over-eighteen crowds (warnings are posted that patrons may not be the age they claim to be).

A women's section is nowhere near as comprehensive, but it may blossom into something more substantial. (Site administrators hint at an eventual spin-off called Jillin' World.) At present, the women's content is limited to information on basic anatomy and masturbation techniques (including using water, dildos, and vibrators to get off). Parents visiting the site are welcomed, reassured, and directed to a good article about the importance of talking to kids about masturbation; a similar welcome greets teens. While most of the site's sex information is quite basic, an "expert" section covers anal stimulation and advanced masturbation techniques. The site's tone is explicit and frank, but it's not intended to be titillating or erotic.

Johan's Guide to Aphrodisiacs

http://www.santesson.com/aphrodis/aphrhome.htm

Forget the popcorn! The next time you take your sweetie to a romantic movie, bring pine nuts along. So suggests the creator of this entertaining encyclopedia of aphrodisiacs. Discover the historical and cultural reasons these fruits, vegetables, herbs, scents, spirits, and animal parts are reputed to have aphrodisiac powers. The site does include a link to the FDA's skeptical stand on aphrodisiacs, but many tips, recipes, and literary references by Johan and other contributors are hard to resist. We suspect there are more than a few people who would be tempted to try this suggestion from the classic Arabic sex manual "The Perfumed Garden": "Drink a glassful of thick honey and eat twenty almonds and one hundred pine nuts before going to bed. After repeating this for three nights, a man will acquire vigor for coition."

The Liberated Christians Homepage

http://www.libchrist.com

United in the belief that people can "lead emotionally and spiritually healthier lives through better sex education and the open discussion of alternative relationship styles," this grassroots polyamory group dishes up a healthy dose of sex information. For example, while the Q&A section addresses common queries about alternative relationships (including how to raise kids in a polyamorous household), it also yields thorough discussions of female ejaculation, oral sex, and anal sex. The fascinating essay on the history of fellatio is accompanied by blow-by-blow instructions on technique. The site includes interpretations of biblical passages related to sexuality.

Meretrix Online

http://www.realm-of-shade.com/meretrix

A legal Nevada prostitute and doctoral student in classical studies, "Mystical Magdalene" is a compelling advocate for the philosophy that sex work is a sacred and valuable profession. Visit her site (*meretrix* is Latin for prostitute) to discover her personally selected online bookshop devoted to issues of commer-

Healthy Sexuality
http://www.healthgate.com/healthy/sexuality
Regular sexual activity (including masturbation) helps regulate menstrual cycles, promotes fertility, increases estrogen in blood and lessens vaginal dryness in post-menopausal women, helps men and women relax better than many pharmaceuticals or alcohol, eases pain in joints and muscles, shields the body from illness and the mind from depression or aggression, promotes a healthy heart, and lengthens life span!

Johan's Guide to Aphrodisiacs
http://www.santesson.com/aphrodis/
aphrhome.htm
Increase sexual vigor by mixing equal parts clarified butter (ghee), honey, sugar, licorice, the juice of fennel bulbs, and milk, into a "nectar-like composition."

Jackin' World
http://www.jackinworld.com
A woman who wants to manually pleasure her partner's penis should remember these mastur-

bation tips: get a good grip, monitor his physical and verbal expressions for cues, ask him what he likes, and don't stop during ejaculation.

Web by Women for Women
http://www.io.com/~wwwomen/queer
In "The Fine Art of Being Come Out To: A Straight Person's Guide to Gay Etiquette," learn what not to say, how to cope with the different situations in which coming out is likely to occur, how to identify potential comings-out and how to make things easier for the outcomer.

Liberated Christians Homepage
http://www.libchrist.org
The delights of fellatio were probably savored even in the dawn of civilization. Many speculate early Middle Easterners learned it by watching domesticated and wild animals licking each other's genitals.

Dr. Eleanor Hamilton
http://www.ptreyeslight.com/columns/
hamilton/hamilton102.html
Advice for the single parent who wants a sex life: "Acknowledge to yourself that you are a sexual being and that your sexuality, when expressed

cial sexuality, sacred prostitution, healing sexuality, and sex magic, as well as a good short set of links related to sex and prostitution. Her FAQ section about her career and her random journal entries make fascinating reading. To the question Why pay for sex? Magdalene answers: "Why pay for someone to cook your food when sharing food is such an intimate thing? Why tithe to a church when spirituality is so sacred? Why pay a psychologist when one should be able to go to one's friends and family for comfort? Courtesans offer more than just pleasure. They offer companionship and an understanding ear."

Museum of Menstruation

http://www.mum.org

What started as one man's fascination with the marketing of feminine hygiene products has evolved into a wacky homage to old Aunt Flo. If lovingly, has a beneficial effect upon every other aspect of your life, including the lives of your children."

Sexual Database
http://www.sexualitydata.com/topics/ fantasy.html
In a study of fifteen thousand women ages eighteen to thirty-four, 97 percent said they fantasize. Most women rely on romantic and erotic fiction or images of past sexual experiences to fuel their fantasy lives.

Elf Sternberg's Hanky FAQ
http://www.halcyon.com/elf/hankies.html
Next time you've a hankering to hump your favorite Hollywood star, wear your silver lamé hanky in your left back pocket. If you see said star wearing the hanky on the right, they're asking for same.

Erotic Vox
http://www.eroticvox.com/ quotes.html
Quotes from famous people throughout history eloquently describe the pleasures of the practice today referred to as BDSM, such as this one from Shakespeare: "Being your slave, what should I do but tend upon the hours and times of your desire?"

Romantic Traveling
http://www.thriveonline.com/sex/travel.htm
Whether you're in the mood for a quick romantic getaway or you need help planning a memorable honeymoon, check out these detailed reviews of inns, cruises, spas, bargain adventures and island destinations.

---

you can navigate the site's confusing design and locate the index of pages, you'll find some wonderful treats. A hodgepodge of articles offer medical, sociological, anthropological, and historical perspectives on menstruation, but the site's crown jewel is its collection of vintage product pamphlets and promotional materials, which have been donated by individuals (such as a tampon salesman's wife) and corporations such as Kotex. View the packaging of the first brand of tampons (known as Fax), which describes them as "internal sanitary napkins," and the glamorous advertisement that scandalized society by using a real woman—a flapper, no less—to sell tampons. You'll find evidence of the museum's somewhat eccentric curator all over the place—he includes material unrelated to menstruation, entries about his cat, Mack C. Padd, and an FAQ section all about himself. You can visit the real museum located in a suburb of Washington, D.C., or take a cybertour on this site.

New Mobility

http://www.newmobility.com

This nicely designed, lively online version of the magazine *New Mobility* is geared toward men and women with physical disabilities. Sex, intimacy, body image, and sexual self-esteem are often addressed in the monthly magazine's feature stories, and a well-maintained archive with search capabilities can help you locate any subject quickly. The magazine devotes one issue each year to the subject of sexuality; the article entitled "Sexual Turning Points" presents a spectrum of readers' peak sexual experiences, including fantasy, cybersex, and the pleasures of giving good head. Visitors can drop in on a regularly scheduled chat about sex (it's in the bar area), post announcements on a discussion board, browse job postings, or peruse recommended readings in the site's bookstore. An extensive link section makes this an excellent gateway resource.

Senior News Network

http://www.seniornews.com

A terrific archive of magazine articles related to seniors. Look in the "Health and Wellness," "Relationships," or "Lifestyles" sections for a smattering of sex information, including an article by Dr. Eleanor Hamilton about the ways in which different prescription drugs can affect your sex life, and another by the author of the best-selling *First Wives Club* about her struggle to gain mainstream acceptance for portrayals of sexy women over the age of fifty.

Sexuality Database

http://www.sexualitydata.com

Billing itself as "The Complete Online Handbook to Sex," this is the closest thing we've seen to an owner's manual for your body and its sexual needs. The brief essays cover the basics of sexual anatomy, health, technique, communication, and various dysfunctions, in addition to harder-to-find material on subjects such as sex and aging and sexual taboos. Explanations sometimes focus on cultural and historical significance at the expense of how-to instruction, but each section is adequately cross-referenced and linked to additional information on other sites. The slight stuffiness of the writing style—for example, "Fellatio is a type of oral sex in which there is mouth contact with the penis"—is predictable given that the text is written by medical professionals. However, the site's vast range of material is presented in a pointedly nonjudgmental and inclusive way, which serves to validate individual sexual experience while encouraging sexual exploration. The site is extremely easy to navigate, thanks in part to the clean design and a handy search function. The *Better Sex* video series is offered for sale since the site is sponsored by the Sinclair Institute, producers of this line of sexual enhancement videos.

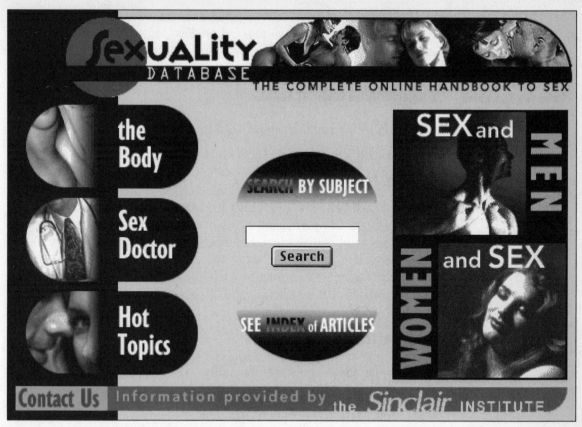

Society for Human Sexuality

http://www.sexuality.org

This granddaddy of sex information sites deserves a place of prominence in your bookmark collection. What started in 1995 as a student project at the University of Washington has blossomed into the biggest online archive of sexuality materials. According to one of the Society's volunteers, the site was "founded on principles of tolerance, open-mindedness, and sex-positivity, with a goal of facilitating basic access to accurate and useful information on all forms of consensual sexuality." The result is an incredibly diverse collection that draws over fifty thousand visitors each month and is on the links list of almost all sex information sites. "A Guide to Caning," "Sexual Positions for Large Lovers," and "How to Pick a Sex Partner" are just a few of the listings in the index, which covers technique, sexual orientation, sexual politics, and regional and national resources. You can download a thorough safer-sex guide and an excellent erotic massage guide at no cost. Society members currently devote significant time to reviewing sex-related books, videos, and products, as well as workshops in the Seattle area. They've also started posting interviews with sex educators.

Understanding Male Sexuality

http://member.aol.com/Sebringsil/sex.htm

Any woman who wants to know what makes her man tick ought to take a look at this site, which offers detailed information about male sexual anatomy and sexual response. Learn which parts of his penis are the most sensitive, teach him how to prolong his arousal and delay ejaculation, and discover why he may particularly enjoy masturbation and fetishes. An excellent discussion of sexual orientation rounds out the site—all that's lacking is more extensive information about the prostate. This site also features a Q&A section about male sexuality, a bibliography, links, and an essay about sex and disability that includes a good discussion of sex toys.

Web by Women for Women

http://www.io.com/~wwwomen/sexuality

On the brink of our first sexual encounters, what wouldn't we have given for this site's essay entitled "Real Live Sex by Real Live People." Perhaps then we wouldn't have expected to kiss dramatically and melt seamlessly into our partners before magically experiencing simultaneous orgasms! This primer will tell you just how to deal with the awkward realities of sex—like what to do when your hair gets in the way, how to get out of an uncomfortable position, how to respond when the penis slips out during intercourse, and how to deal with cleanup. It's just one essay on a wonderful site devoted to the effect of censorship on women's sexuality, which also includes sections on contraception, pregnancy, menstruation, and sexual preferences. The small group of women behind the site deliver some great rants (despite the occasional lapse into rhetoric), and they welcome reader feedback and contributions. Find out what other women think about their sexual entertainment options, listen to a sixty-year-old woman's request to be seen as a sexual being, read up on some erotic fan fiction (in which *The X-Files's* Mulder and Scully finally do it), link to pictures of "yummy" naked men, share stories about losing your virginity, or read advice for the woman on the brink of losing hers. While the site primarily represents heterosexual women, lesbian participation is enthusiastically encouraged, and women of any sexual preference will appreciate the abundance of real stories about real women's sexual desires.

Womb

http://womb.wwdc.com

All too many lesbian resource sites suffer from the "Where's the sex?" syndrome, but this one's an exception. Buried amid the extensive list of links to lesbian sites (including lesbian erotica, art, and e-zines) are valuable, if brief, guides to female ejaculation and vaginal fisting along with a positive discussion of S/M. The author's occasional preference for stream-of-consciousness writing can be distracting (how many ellipses can you put in one sentence?) and the sex information is served up with a bit of lesbian-feminist rhetoric (webmistress Kelly Garland waxes on about the patriarchy, oppression, and heterosexual evils). But if you think the author takes herself too seriously, check out the "Authentic Lesbian Manifesto"—a tongue-in-cheek look at politically correct lesbianism, from which we can't resist quoting: "All Authentic Lesbians must never admit to PD (Penetration Desire). This includes the desire to be penetrated by a dildo, or by a woman wearing a strap-on dildo or any other sex toy which even remotely resembles a penis. Any Authentic Lesbian discovered to be 'packing' will be subject to public interrogation by members of the local ALC. If penetration is absolutely essential, it is suggested that vegetables be used instead. Preferably those shaped to resemble the form of a short, overweight goddess, a bunny, a cat, a whale, or k.d. lang. Jodie Foster is permitted, but only in her 'butchier' mode." The site also features rotating exhibits of contemporary erotic art.

World Sex Guide—Prostitution Around the World

http://www.worldsexguide.com

The alt.sex.prostitution newsgroup started out as a way for guys to swap information about where to get laid. They've archived so much material that the resulting Web site reads kind of like a *Michelin Guide* to prostitution around the world. Not only do they review brothels, bars, clubs, massage parlors, escort services, call girls, and street prostitutes—they also discuss the legal situation, enforcement policies, and working environment in different cities. Sex workers post advertisements and information as well, and the site features a search service, newsletter, glossary, and links to great resources. For a real treat, we recommend checking out a few of these guys' narratives—they provide great fantasy fuel as well as fascinating insight into the male libido. The authors describe their site this way: "There are no ads, pictures, graphics, sounds or Java applets on this site. No flashing colors and blinking shit either. We don't need that stuff, because we have information instead."

The Body: Safe Sex and Prevention

http://www.thebody.com/safesex.html

Articles and information about safer sex culled from a wide variety of sources (medical journals, the Centers for Disease Control, Planned Parenthood, health sites) are posted here, conveniently categorized by issues relevant to gay men, women, teens, health care workers, and drug users. In addition, you'll find links to general safer-sex instruction, a FAQ section, vaccine updates, a list of HIV hotlines, and advice about everything from how to improve the taste of oral sex with condoms to how to tell a partner you're infected. Maintained by Rick Sowadsky, the coordinator for the Nevada AIDS Hotline, who has over a decade of experience in HIV education and counseling.

Contraceptive Guide

http://www.mjbovo.com/contracep.htm

A straightforward guide to the varieties of contraception currently available, presented by Doctor Mary Jane Bovo, known as the "Ann Landers of the gynecological world." She clearly compares effectiveness rates, costs, and the advantages and disadvantages of every birth control method from the pill and condoms to sponges and natural family-planning methods. Don't miss the refresher course on conception, a gentle reminder that withdrawal, sex during one's period, and praying are all ineffective methods!

Healthy Sexuality

http://www.healthgate.com/healthy/sexuality

Regular visits to this online magazine will benefit your sex life as much as a good fitness regimen benefits your health. Lively, timely articles written by health professionals and journalists cover an impressive array of subjects related to sex and relationships. New material appears weekly to keep you abreast of matters that affect your sexual health, including the latest on STDs, the relationship between nutrition and your libido, the effect prescription drugs have on your sex life, and when and why you might consider sex therapy. You'll also find discussions of more specific sexual problems, such as impotence, painful sex, and various disabilities. Sexual enhancement gets equal time in articles on fantasy, mutual masturbation, tantric sex, and rekindling desire, as do interviews with sex-positive luminaries such as Nancy Friday, Dr. Ruth, and Joycelyn Elders. Articles are cross-referenced to others in the "Healthy Living" series—a collection of online magazines that address men's health, women's health, parenting, and nutrition.

Naked Truth About STDs

http://www.unspeakable.com

This frank, accurate, and unabashed guide to the prevention and treatment of sexually transmitted diseases does not include the explicit photos you may find on other STD pages. It offers medical information and practical personal resources, such as a list of questions to ask your doctor and tips for talking with partners (with sample dialogues). Based on the input you provide about your sexual history, the "risk profiler" assesses your overall risk level and offers suggestions for modifying your behavior. You can also take an STD quiz, brush up on basic information at the site's FAQ section, and use the "clinic locator" to find a clinic near you. Created by a pharmaceutical company with the participation of a doctor from the Centers for Disease Control, the site is professionally presented and easy to navigate.

Safer Sex Page

http://www.safersex.org

Are condoms reusable? How do I get one out of the wrapper without tearing it? Where can I buy them? What is lubricant? Answers to these and other safer-sex questions can be found on this friendly, comprehensive site, which takes a creative approach to sex education. Multimedia bells and whistles such as a video visit to a condom factory, cartoons illustrating condom use, and audio tips from couples practicing safer-sex negotiation make this site a must-visit for people of all ages and sexual preferences. Parents will find tips for raising their child's comfort level with the language of sex, as well as pointers on how to get their kids to buy condoms. It's all here— information on risk management, lesbian sex, female condoms, birth control, and STDs—along with the promise of a Q&A section, a chat room, and a quarterly magazine.

Nothing aggravates parents more than kids whining "Are we there yet?" from the backseat of the family car. Now we can all experience the same pain and frustration as those kids as we travel the byways of the Web. How many of us sit idly in front of our computers waiting for a page to load and wondering, "Am I there yet?"—only to despair when the answer is No! No! No! Here are a few of the most annoying speed bumps that conspire to slow us down:

Intermediary pages. After browsing the table of contents, you click on the title of an article you'd like to read and wait the requisite minute or so for the accompanying graphic to materialize, only to discover that you've arrived at yet another page with the same title (and perhaps a short blurb about the piece), which you then must click to get to the actual article. Why not go directly to the article? Beats us!

To be continued. We understand the value of a "to be continued" or "more" button when it appears at the bottom of a page containing an abundance of text or product illustrations—after all, it's important not to overcrowd the screen. However, we have noticed heavy abuse of the "more" button in commercial sites, in which, for example, a selection of product photos might get parceled out three at a time. Imagine having to walk down a different aisle in the drug store every time you wanted to see three more bottles of shampoo! We'd like to see a larger selection at one time; it is not only less time-consuming but also makes it easier to comparison shop. The best sites offer thumbnail images, which load up quickly, along with the option of choosing which thumbnails the viewer would like to see enlarged.

Counterintuitive names for links. You're on the homepage and you want to read about the site's creators or company mission. Odds are good that headings like "About Us" and "Company Philosophy" will get you where you want to go, but in an effort to differentiate their sites, some designers come up with desperately clever, unhelpful names such as "Town Hall" or "Workings." Off you go, only to hit the Back button again and again as you repeatedly find yourself in the wrong place. In keeping with the driving metaphors so popular on the information superhighway, that's what we'd call a lousy road map.

Sexual Health Infocenter

http://www.sexhealth.org/infocenter

A fairly comprehensive and upbeat collection of sex advice and information, with an emphasis on sex toy how-tos because of the site's affiliation with the Renaissance online catalog (see p. 141). You'll find basic facts about STDs and safer sex (including a welcome essay on "making it fun"), as well as practical tips for enhancing sex. We were impressed by the coverage of less–commonly addressed topics such as sex and aging, and sexual dysfunctions, as well as a lengthy description of sexual positions, with certain ones recommended for the mobility impaired. The

Q&A column "Ask Renaissance" is frequently updated, but the laundry list of over a year's worth of questions is hard to navigate (this is somewhat remedied by a search function). Visitors are invited to participate in quarterly surveys of sexual activities; the results are posted. Overall, the information is sound, but periodically, women's sexuality gets short shrift—the absence of any mention of the female condom and the annoying generalizations about lesbian sexuality are surprising given the excellent discussions of safer sex, vibrators, and dildos in other sections. Apparently the site is the product of consultations with a host of unnamed health professionals, but we found it difficult to learn much about the authors or their advisors.

Sexual Health Network

http://www.sexualhealth.com

If you're disabled, finding any information pertinent to your sex life presents a formidable challenge, and the Web is one of the best places to look. Created by Michael Pepper, a Ph.D. student who suffered a spinal cord injury, the site presents information compiled on sexual issues specific to an extensive (though not exhaustive) list of mental or physical disabilities, including options for erectile dysfunction, advice for women interested in intercourse, suggestions for physically negotiating sexual activities, and information about fertility, adoption, parenting, and contraception. Articles in the "Love Bites" section cover more general issues such as sex toys, self-esteem, dating, sexual positions, desire issues, sensate focus, and enjoying sex after an injury. This site also offers sex-ed training programs for individuals, educators, and health professionals. Book recommendations and links to other disability sites round out this incredible resource.

STD Homepage

http://med-www.bu.edu/people/sycamore/std

Learn the cause, incubation period, symptoms, and treatment for a variety of sexually transmitted diseases and conditions, including AIDS, chlamydia, gonorrhea, hepatitis B, herpes, pubic lice, syphilis, and venereal warts. A glossary of terms improves reader comprehension immensely, but there is not much information about behavior or risk management. You will need a strong stomach to view the graphic photos of oozing lesions and bloody scabs, but they come in handy if you're trying to identify an STD.

alt.sex.column

http://www.sfbg.com/asc

Buckle your seat belts! Based on the range of sexual activities covered in this Q&A column—which promises "sex education for the new millennium"—we're taking the fast lane into the twenty-first century. In her *San Francisco Bay Guardian* online column, Andrea Nemerson fields the usual round of anatomy questions but also covers an impressive range of alternative sexual activities, including threesomes, swinging, BDSM, anal sex, vaginal fisting, and dildo play (providing helpful links to other sites in the process). Nemerson, a longtime volunteer and trainer at the San Francisco Sex Information Switchboard, claims to have answered over two thousand questions about sex in her day and promises "not to think you're weird for asking. If I haven't done it myself, I'll either find someone who has or give you a good reason why you shouldn't either." The *Guardian* site offers a cumbersome search service, a shame since the questions are often titled ambiguously. For all you beach bunnies visiting or living in California, check out the impressive guide to nude beaches (accompanied by Phyllis Christopher's nude photographs), located elsewhere on the *Guardian* site.

Ask Delilah

http://thriveonline.com/passion.html

Have you ever longed for a trusted aunt or older sister who could give you sex advice laced with affection and good humor? Health educator Delilah (formerly of Go Ask Alice!; see p. 104) is the next-best thing—her "Ask Delilah" column is infused with enthusiasm, encouragement, and warmth. As the resident sexpert for the *Thrive Passion* site, she advises readers on both common and seldom-discussed issues related to sex and relationships, from advice on what to give your boyfriend for Valentine's Day to how to deal with the "wet spot." We especially appreciate the column's cross-referencing feature, which lists related questions alongside each Q&A. While the archives—filled with hundreds of past Q&As—would benefit from categorization, a useful search function will put you in touch with the information you desire.

Don't limit your visit to the advice section. *Thrive Passion* also contains a range of short articles on birth control, relationship issues (e.g., "Monogamy Vs. Monotony," "Is Cybersex Cheating?"), general sex information on topics ranging from tantric sex to ejaculation control to "The Key to Kinky

Happiness," and an excellent series of links to STD-related sites. The bustling (should we say thriving?) message boards deal with a great range of sexual topics, are open to all, and are easy to read and post to. *Thrive* is an online health and fitness magazine that is part of Time Warner's monolithic Pathfinder site. We could live without the *Cosmo*-style polls and quizzes ("Are You a Flirt?"), but that's the price you pay for corporate sponsorship. On the flip side, the advantage of such sponsorship is the site's readability, ease of use, and general professionalism; new material goes up daily.

Ask Me Anything

http://www.sexed.org

Sex therapist Marty Klein's Q&A column features over two dozen questions on topics from the effects of antidepressants on one's sex life to concerns about sexual incompatibility. The questions on his site are excerpted from his book, *Ask Me Anything,* which is for sale on the site. Klein also posts some of his other writing, both mainstream magazine articles and professional papers in which he tackles the subject of cybersex (is it sex?), muses on the talk-show phenomenon, and explains why there's no such thing as sex addiction.

Ask The Couch!

http://www.askthecouch.com

This is one of our favorite Q&A sites—not just because the authors, married hipsters named Thomas and Courtney, answered our own (anonymous) question in a timely manner but because their sex advice comes with equal parts humor, candor, and thoughtfulness. Some might find the humor a little in-your-face, but that's what makes the site entertaining as well as informative. They tackle an amazing variety of subjects, including fetishes, choosing a dildo, penis size, genital shaving tips, sexual fantasies, and clit jewelry. Their accurate, thorough answers are well linked to further resources. Columns are archived chronologically, with annotated descriptions of the subjects addressed within each listing. An adults-only chat room is also featured.

Dr. Ruth Online

http://www.drruth.com

If you like your sex information delivered in bite-sized nuggets by a well-known, grandmotherly sex educator, visit Doctor Ruth's site. She answers dozens of sex questions grouped into three main categories: teens, adults, and seniors. Her advice is usually sound, but her safer-sex information is substandard and downbeat. She updates the site regularly with sex tips and short musings on sexual enhancement (including a reassuring statement about cross-dressing), provides a fascinating brief autobiography, and includes an excellent bibliography of books and videos. Clear, crisp graphics suit the doc's quirky, no-nonsense, encouraging style.

In a bizarre merger of sex, technology, and marketing, Dr. Ruth features a page of "desktop goodies," from which you can download little icons or background patterns depicting everything from the female condom to art from the *Kama Sutra!* In case you'd like a more personal connection, you can listen to audio snippets of Dr. Ruth reciting her tips—but good luck keeping a straight face!

Go Ask Alice!

http://www.goaskalice.columbia.edu

You've got a burning sex question and you just can't bring yourself to ask your best friend or your doctor. Now you can join the thousands of other curious folks (mostly college students) who log on each week to read Alice's answers to queries about everything from self-esteem to birth control to sexual technique. Maintained by Columbia University, this site evolved out of the need to provide accurate, frank, and honest information to its student population and now boasts one of the most extensive archives of sex Q&As available online. The fictional Alice (a team of health educators) addresses issues of general emotional and physical health, but the sexuality and relationship sections receive the lion's share of activity. The site's search function is essential, since the long lists of questions are simply categorized under the broad topics of sexual health, sexuality, and relationships. Unfortunately, the search button doesn't appear on the Q&A page, so you need to go through an extra step or two to find your information (tip: go into the "Healthwise" option and select "Interactive Alice"). This could well be the most exhaustive sex Q&A online.

Self-Help and Psychology Q&A

http://www.cybertowers.com/selfhelp/qa

Unique to this site is a special section devoted to questions about cyber-sex (What is it? Is it addictive?), which help demystify this increasingly popular practice. In the "Sex and Lust" section, sex therapist Al Cooper pro-

FREE-FLOWING ADVICE

In the '90s Ann Landers answered a question about masturbation in her syndicated advice column and jaws dropped all across the country. Some folks took issue with her comments (which were pro-masturbation), but many people were simply shocked by the fact that there, in broad daylight, a national guardian of etiquette was waxing about wanking!

For those of you who'd rather not hold your breath waiting for the likes of Ann or Abby to drop a sexual pearl of wisdom, the Web offers a host of advice columns, in which "sexperts" dispense frank and accurate sex information on nearly every conceivable wrinkle. In fact, with so many to choose from, you can shop around for the advisor whose personality and style suit you best. Whether you want your advice sprinkled with medical terms, peppered with sarcasm, or overflowing with reassurances, there's a doctor, a hipster, or the equivalent of a sex-savvy older sister ready to oblige you online.

As a way of illustrating various styles, we're quoting from a few of the advice columnists who appear on sites reviewed in this book. We chose anal sex as our subject because women and men are enjoying this activity in greater numbers than ever before; because it's easily one of the most popular sex topics online; and because it's not a topic the mainstream media covers. We're quite certain even Ann Landers won't be venturing into this territory anytime soon!

Isadora Alman's Sexuality Forum
http://www.askisadora.com
Isadora Alman, M.A., is a board-certified sexologist, California licensed relationship counselor, author, and nationally syndicated columnist ("Ask Isadora"). She doesn't take questions on her site (see p. 178), which is devoted to a community discussion board, but the site does include a well-organized archive of excerpts from her print column.

Q: *What percentage of women out there enjoy anal sex, and what physiological reason could explain a pleasurable or orgasmic feeling from this experience? Bottom line, are there any out there who really desire and dig it, and why?*

A: Bottom line? I can't quote statistics, however there is a much larger percentage of women who enjoy receiving oral sex than anal, basically because there is a greater likelihood of their achieving orgasm by clitoral stimulation than anal or rectal. Men (gay, straight and bi) have a bonus inducement for such stimulation in their prostate, although all genders and orientations have many nerve endings around the anus which can respond positively. There are women who do enjoy anal sex and who might give you a variety of reasons why, but fundamentally (oh dear!), people become sexually aroused (some to the point of orgasm) by what feels good to them, whether there is a clitoris in the vicinity or not.

alt.sex.column
http://www.sfbg.com/asc
Andrea Nemerson writes this column for the online edition of the weekly *San Francisco Bay Guardian*. She volunteers and trains at the San Francisco Sex Information Switchboard (415–989–7374 or http://www.sfsi.org).

Q: *My girlfriend and I want to try anal sex. Fantasies about it really turn us on. We've tried a couple times but it was always pretty painful for her. Is there a "best" position for it?*

A: Rear-approach seems to make sense for rear-entry, but the operative concepts here are actually control and freedom of movement. On hands and knees, your girlfriend can scoot forward or back at will. It has been demonstrated that people fear flying far more than driving, although cars are far more likely to kill you. However imperiled, a driver feels like the captain of her own fate, which will tend to assuage fears of the unknown and uncontrollable. No fear, no muscle tension, no pain. Let her drive. *Continued*

Anal insertion of anything requires patience, trust, and copious quantities of store-bought lube. Spit simply won't do. Start—slowly—with a well-manicured finger. Keep talking, build up gradually, and stop immediately or sooner at the first twinge of fear or discomfort.

The really great thing about bungholes, of course, is that everybody has one. "I don't know how it feels, so how can I do it right?" will not get you out of this one. The best way to learn how to penetrate a nervous beginner is to be one. Hand her the lube, me bucko, and assume the position.

Ask the Couch!
http://www.askthecouch.com
Thomas and Courtney are a married couple who vigorously pooh-pooh the idea that anyone needs a credential to offer advice on the topic of sexual relationships (but she's an M.D. and he's a registered counselor with a B.A. in psychology).

Q: Me and my boyfriend have tried anal sex and succeeded, on several occasions. I really enjoyed it and would like to do it again. My question is why, if I enjoy it, is it still painful?

A: Anal sex is like everything else in life, if it is painful, don't do it! Since you have had successful butt sex, it's obviously not a hang-up for you but you're not a pro yet either. It takes some practice and a little research and planning for a bout of rear entry! The number one rule of anal sex is if it starts to hurt, stop all action (you don't have to withdraw) RELAX . . . TAKE . . . SOME . . . DEEP . . . BREATHS, and continue slowly, maintaining maximum comfort thus pleasure. Your homework for tonight's class is to read the rest of the "Ten Rules of Anal Sex" [author Jack Morin's excellent tips, reprinted on the Good Vibrations Web site; see p. 134].

Self-Help and Psychology Q&A
http://www.cybertowers.com/selfhelp/qa
Al Cooper, Ph.D., is a sex therapist and psychology professor who writes the "Sex and Lust" column for this online magazine.

Q: Don't you have to be sick or weird to have or want anal sex?

A: It is fairly common for people to have strong reactions around the subject of anal sex—that is, sexual activity that involves stimulating the anorectal area—often because of shame as well as anxiety around homosexuality that is thought to be associated with it. However, artifacts depicting anal intercourse found in Incan ruins indicate that this variant of sexual practice was known in antiquity. Apparently, the practice is not only known but fairly common in the United States today. Studies reveal that it is most common among homosexual men and least common among lesbians. In the vast middle, 22–43% of bisexual and heterosexual men and women report that they have tried it at least once.

Anal sex is not for every one—even male homosexuals. Different studies indicate that anal sex is not the primary preferred method of sexual activity even for gay men. So it is hard to generalize about who would enjoy this activity and who would not. That's part of what makes sexuality novel and exciting—exploring what works best for you and your partner. Remember that there are "different strokes for different folks." No one should feel pressured into doing something they are not comfortable with nor should someone be judged for liking something other than mainstream sex.

Ask Dr. Myrtle
http://www.a-womans-touch.com
Myrtle Wilhite, M.D., M.S., co-owns A Woman's Touch sexuality store.

Q: Doesn't the desire for anal penetration say something about my sexual orientation?

A: Nerve endings do not understand about "orientation." Nerve endings respond to sensory stimuli (touch, taste, sound, etc.) while only whole people get involved with cultural messages about who "should" love or be intimate with whom. If someone likes to be intimate in certain areas of their body, it means nothing about their orientation, past, present, or future.

Anal eroticism fascinates many people, whether in fantasy or reality. Some of the basis for this may be related to the high number of sensory nerve endings dedicated to sensation surrounding the anus and skin in the perianal region (skin surrounding the anus).

vides thorough, upbeat answers to questions on loss of desire, sex toys, and taboos. More health and relationship information can be found in the "Teens" and "Gays and Lesbians" categories. New questions are posted regularly, but there is neither a search function nor a topical breakdown of subjects.

Sex Clinic with Dr. Patti Britton

http://www.sexclinic.com

Sex therapist and co-founder of Feminists for Free Expression (see p. 207), Dr. Patti Britton dispenses thorough information in a nonjudgmental way and refers readers to a variety of toys, videos, and books (her site is sponsored by a sex toy company). Questions in the Sex Clinic are conveniently organized by topic and address issues ranging from desire discrepancy to orgasm 101 to golden showers. If you can't find the answer to your question in the clinic's archives, you can query Dr. Britton by e-mail or phone for a fee. The heart of the clinic lies in the "Confessionals" page, where readers write in about favorite fantasies, turn-ons, and sexual dilemmas. Unlike the *Penthouse* letters style of fabricated confessions, these genuinely reflect the vast spectrum of sexual experience and fantasy (Who could make up the one about Popeye?). Britton's news updates about matters related to health and sexuality will keep you well informed.

Women's Wire Sexperts

http://www.womenswire.com

One of the oldest and most comprehensive women's online directories, Women's Wire puts viewers in touch with everything from investment advice to soap opera updates. It also features a "Love and Sex" Q&A, hosted by sex educator Patrizia DiLucchio (we love her for mentioning a Hitachi Magic Wand in her profile) and Andy Erdman, a TV scriptwriter and college instructor. Their columns are separate, so you must choose whether to submit your question to her (in "Ask Sexpert") or him (in "Ask eMale"). Sexpert's tone is sensible and occasionally humorous, but eMale's tone tends toward flip and clever at the expense of providing useful feedback. Still, he's worth a visit to get the average Joe's perspective on breast implants, faking orgasm, threesomes, or getting out of a sexual rut. Overall, these columns focus more on relationships than sex, and the sexual content is erratic: it was gratifying to see information about how piercings enhance erotic experience, but disappointing to find nothing on anal sex. The convenient search function makes up for a format that suffers from the "Are we there yet?" syndrome.

Chapter Five

Parenting and Sex Education

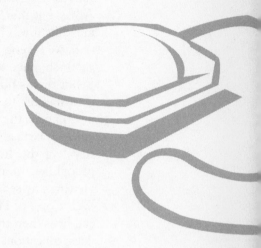

The ABCs of Sex Ed

Did you see the episode of *Sesame Street* in which Big Bird teaches kids about sexual anatomy? He lifts up a baby muppet's dress to reveal her anatomically correct genitals. "Now, boys and girls, we're going to look at little Maggie's clitoris," he says. Grover, Cookie Monster, and Maria gather round and sing a song about the clitoris, and by the end of the show everyone knows what C stands for.

Okay, it didn't really happen, but we can dream, can't we? We're among the many adults who believe that teaching children about sex should come just as naturally and comfortably as educating them about everything else in their young lives. If our kids learn about noses and toes from Big Bird, why shouldn't they learn the names of *all* the parts of the body? By omitting this information, we not only miss an opportunity to teach them that sexuality is good; we actually give them their first message that it's not—a message they will receive countless times in their lives.

Even the most well-intentioned, best-prepared parents struggle with sex education. I, Anne, have an eighteen-month-old daughter who likes to rub her plastic Winnie the Pooh figurines against her labia during bath time.

After ten years of working in the field of sex education, I know that this is a perfectly normal activity. And while I would never stop her, I still have trouble taking advantage of this golden opportunity to rehearse the names of her genitals—something I do instinctively when she's playing with the other parts of her body.

I often wish for a little help from the usual sources. Christopher Robin's gang teaches my daughter about friendship, and Big Bird helps with her ABCs, but there's no way she'll ever see Barney talking about kiddie genitalia like it was just another walk in the park. When it comes to sex education, we parents are on our own. Unfortunately, most of us don't do a very good job, since we didn't get any decent sex education either.

But there's hope in sight—I mean, site. The Web can make a significant contribution to your child's sex education. You probably haven't heard much about the Web's potentially positive effect on a child's sexual development, because this good news has been overshadowed by the media portrayal of the Internet as a dangerous zone filled with pornography and pedophiles. In all the hoopla over finding ways to "protect" our kids from viewing any sexually explicit material online (see the sidebar "Don't Be a Web Cop," p. 112), few have noted what a priceless sex resource the Web can be. When the subject is *not* sex, everyone agrees that there are tremendous educational and interactive opportunities for kids online—toddlers can color pictures of Big Bird or have stories read to them, preteens can get help with their math homework, and teens can write, edit, and publish their own zines. It should come as no surprise, then, that this same technology can be used to help kids learn about their sexuality, as well as to give parents and teachers the tools to teach kids about sex.

What the Web Can Do for You

The following are some ways in which the Web can help you.

Improve Your Own Sexual Literacy

Most people agree that parents should be responsible for their children's sex education, but what happens when a parent's own sexual literacy falls painfully short? By visiting any one of the many excellent sex information sites online, you can answer your own sex questions, which will put you in a much better position to answer your child's. Expanding your knowledge of sexual issues expands your own comfort level, which in turn should make talking with your kids a lot less awkward. What's more, since you can access sites from around the world, you may broaden your understanding of sex by learning how it is experienced in other cultures. And by viewing as many sites as you can, you will be well equipped to create a comprehensive list of sex education sites suitable for your child.

Be Prepared

Your six-year-old daughter bursts into your bedroom while you and your partner are making love. If you've visited any of the "how to talk to your kids about sex" sites, you'll resist the urge to banish her abruptly from the room and never speak about what happened. Many of these sites offer practice dialogue and loads of advice to help you prepare for each stage of your child's sexual development. Considering that kids enter this world as sexual beings, it's never too early to learn how to answer those surprise questions sensitively or how to initiate a discussion about a sexual issue. By doing so you contribute to your child's sexual self-esteem and create a comfortable environment for future dialogue.

Call in the Cavalry

Schools and teachers play an important part in the sexual upbringing of today's youth. A recent poll by Planned Parenthood revealed that 82 percent of Americans favor sex education in schools and that the majority prefer more comprehensive programs, rather than those that just advocate abstinence. And although most people believe that parents should be responsible for their child's sex education, only 7 percent of those polled by *Time* magazine had actually learned about sex from their own parents. Teachers and counselors are often thrust into the role of substitute parents—called upon to provide sex information when a child is unable to confide in a parent. All students deserve consistent, accurate information, and all teachers deserve the benefit of training. Organizations such as SIECUS and Planned Parenthood offer strategies on their Web sites for developing a sex education curriculum that goes well beyond reproductive information and for dealing with potential concerns raised by administrators and parents.

Give Your Child Resources

Elsewhere in this book we've lauded the Web as a place where people can find both vital resources and a community of like-minded people. These are two important reasons to give your child access to sexual materials online. You may feel that your child can talk to you about anything, but he or she may feel differently. You can't afford to wait around and hope your children will ask you about sex; instead, let them know there are other ways to get the information. The Web hosts some extraordinary sites offering information about everything from puberty to safer sex to sexual technique, many written in a language and style accessible to kids.

As soon as the Supreme Court declared that the Communications Decency Act was an unconstitutional effort to "protect" children from "indecent" materials on the Internet, scores of politicians, parents' groups, and high-tech organizations announced their intention to work together toward a common goal: limiting kids' access to sexually explicit materials online. And the tool these coalitions most commonly endorse is filtering (also known as blocking) software. Filtering programs such as CyberSitter, CyberPatrol, SurfWatch, and others work in conjunction with your browser to block access to sites containing "adult" material; the filters block sites either by searching the software's list of banned sites or by searching for certain keywords and phrases.

Filtering software is just the latest example of how hard we try to keep kids from seeing or knowing much about sex. Despite evidence to the contrary, we fear that if we let little Joey look at *Playboy* he might grow up to be a pervert, or if Sally finds out what a penis looks like she might turn into a nymphomaniac. As a society, our approach to sex education can be characterized as evasive and restrictive, all in the name of protecting our children. Unfortunately, this practice runs contrary to our kids' natural desires to explore their sexuality and seek answers to the questions that can help them make responsible choices concerning their sexual health. Ultimately, our efforts often harm the children we hope to protect, as evidenced by the ever-rising rates of teen pregnancy, gay suicide, and STD transmission among youth.

Knowledge is power, and children have just as much right to both as adults do. That's why we don't support legislation that seeks to regulate content on the Web or software designed to block access to "questionable" sites. We certainly won't argue that there's no such thing as tasteless porn online (we wouldn't be writing this book if that were the case), but we feel that children should be encouraged to discuss material that makes them uncomfortable or curious. These discussions give parents the opportunity to convey critical information and to communicate their own values. As one of our survey respondents states succinctly, "If the lines of communication between me and my kids are not open enough for us to talk about what they see online,

Based on the popularity of several of these sites, it appears that the Web is the only source many young adults have for accurate sex information. Go Ask Alice!, a question-and-answer site maintained by Columbia University, receives over two hundred questions each week and reports one million visitors annually. The Coalition for Positive Sexuality (CPS), a nonprofit that typically distributes about five hundred hard copies a week of its safer-sex booklet, *Just Say Yes*, now reaches one thousand teens each day on its Web page. Both sites serve visitors from all over the world.

The high traffic on these sites underscores the inadequacy of traditional sex education methods. System administrators marvel over the level of naiveté in teenagers and college students. Anaheed Alani, the Q&A person at CPS, says that the number-one reason teens seek out the site is to find out if they're pregnant. "Lots of kids are getting little or no information about birth control," she says. "They use the withdrawal and rhythm then we have bigger problems than a simple 'search on penis.'" Another parent explains her reasons for rejecting filters: "I treat the Web as I would films, books, or radio. If my daughter sees an erotic image that intrigues her, she always asks me about it. It's more difficult to explain war crime photographs to your child than it is to explain what people are doing having intercourse, which is a snap by comparison."

We understand why filtering software may sound appealing—and why you might prefer to bypass the seamier side of the Web entirely—but its application is problematic. We sincerely hope that after reading our tips on using the Web to enhance your child's sex education, you'll log on and visit some of the suggested sites. But if you're using filtering software, there's a good chance that many of the sites we've recommended will be inaccessible, for any number of reasons. If your software blocks sites based on sex-related key words, it won't necessarily discriminate between sex education and porn. Your software's rating criteria may classify masturbation or homosexuality as unacceptable topics. Even if your software includes ratings for tens of thousands of sites, it may block access to hundreds of thousands of sites that haven't been rated yet.

If you still feel you want to use filtering software, please take the time to research which one you select. Find out what criteria the company uses to block sites, who rates sites for them, how many sites they have rated to date, and to what extent you can customize the filtering to reflect your own values. Most companies refuse to provide a list of the sites their software blocks, but many online free-speech organizations publish this information (see chapter 9, "Free Speech and the Future," for information on these organizations).

Call us Pollyannas, but we have high hopes that parents, librarians, teachers, and kids can use the Web to improve communication about a variety of sensitive topics and enjoy a rich learning experience in the process. We couldn't agree more with Victoria Williams, author of *Internet for Kids*: "I firmly believe that if we teach our young people the positive uses of the media and communication technologies, they will make the best of them. They will also know how to bring moral values, good taste and logical judgment to what they read and believe."

For more information about filtering software, see chapter 9 or visit Peacefire (see p. 209), an anticensorship site created by teens.

methods, but no one has told them they're not safe." From what she's seen, kids get a basic biology lesson in school, but that's where any sexual discussion ends. There is no explicit talk about physical and sexual pleasure. "It's sad that they could know how reproduction happens, but not how orgasms happen. And that they seem to know more about how babies are made than they do about masturbation."

Community can be just as critical to teens. As CPS webmaster Brad Borevitz says, "Imagine the relief when a scared, gay kid from some backwater town goes online and finds not only other gay kids to talk to, but kids who couldn't care less about his orientation." The anonymity of online chat emboldens teens to say what's really on their minds, resulting in a free-flowing forum of frank talk on a variety of topics. Participants educate, encourage, advise, and often tolerate one another in a way that's not possible in the real world, where peer groups are small and equally ill-informed, where school sex talks are limited to clinical discussions of disease prevention, and where most parents would recoil in horror at a question about fellatio technique.

Now that we've given you plenty of reasons to get yourself and your kids online, we hope you'll use the sites recommended in the reviews section as your jumping-off point.

How to Make the Web Even Better

Although the exceptional sites we review here deliver good sex information to parents and kids, the bad news is that the state of online sex education could be vastly improved. Quality and access are the two main problem areas.

For example, while there are some noteworthy youth-friendly sex sites, there aren't any sites for young children. You can access a *Sesame Street* site that will read stories aloud to your kids, but this technology is never extended to that classic story, "How Babies Are Made." Designers are understandably cautious about creating sex education sites with engaging graphics for fear of crossing the line between what is educational and what is perceived to be exploitative or even pornographic. Content is similarly compromised in sites for older children. Any good book about puberty or adolescence will contain anatomically correct illustrations, but these images are very hard to come by online. Why? Nobody wants to risk being labeled a child pornographer!

Even those sex education sites that exist can be extremely hard to find. General interest sites for preteens and adolescents—which ideally would link to the best sex education sites—won't touch sexual topics with a ten-foot pole. The popular kids' directory Yahooligans produces absolutely no matches for searches on "puberty" or "sex education." Ideally, parents will have the patience and persistence to track down good sites (our recommendations should get you started) and bookmark these for their kids.

What can you do about this state of affairs? Defend your child's right to good sex education by exploring the resources of the Web together, rather than relying on the false security of filtering softwares that will block access to valuable sex information. Teach your children safe surfing habits (see the sidebar on p. 119), and encourage their powers of discrimination. You can ensure a safe journey online by teaching them not to give out personal information and to question—and report back to you—any online encounters that make them uncomfortable.

And while you're at it, we'd encourage you to speak up in defense of sex information online. Support the good sites you've found, and steer your fellow parents toward them. Why not write to the Children's Television Network and tell them it's time for Big Bird to explain all about the clitoris and the penis in an online storybook? Next time you're in a parenting chat room or discussion board and you can't find any sex topics listed, offer to start a topic or two yourself. Many sites will appreciate and encourage your initiative. After all, the Web is what we make it.

Reviews

PARENTS AND TEACHERS

Circumcision Information Page

http://www.cirp.org

To circumcise or not? If that is your question, you must check out the Circumcision Information Page before the little tyke is born. You'll find an abundance of information, including answers to parents' frequently asked questions, articles about medical, cultural, and religious issues, foreskin restoration advice, readers' comments, and numerous useful illustrations. The discussion of the foreskin's role in sexual enjoyment is particularly enlightening.

CyberMom Pillow Talk

http://www.TheCyberMom.com

Hey moms, ever wonder what other parents do when the kiddies interrupt their lovemaking? Interested in how they decided whether or not to circumcise their sons? Looking for a few creative, inexpensive ways to seduce your mate? Visit the "Pillow Talk" or "Powder Room" (dealing with health issues) in CyberMom's easy-to-navigate floor plan and you'll find discussion boards about dozens of topics related to sexuality. Among the hundreds of topics posted by moms, many focus on broader relationship issues, but you will find a variety of sex discussions, ranging from Internet infidelity to desire discrepancies. However, since participants have so many topics to choose from (and probably so little free time!), the discussions can be quite short.

This site is a great place to gab with your peers about sex, but if you're looking for comprehensive answers to specific sex questions, you should visit one of our recommended sex information sites.

Hip Mama

http://www.hipmama.com

Nope, *Hip Mama* is not the cheap attention-getting moniker of an amateur porn star. It's the quarterly zine devoted to "straight talk and good humor about the joys and craziness of parenting." *Hip Mama's* Web site contains the same rants, reviews, and classifieds as the paper zine, but the *Hip Mama* conference boards and chat room provide one of the few opportunities—on- or offline—for women and men to share information about how their sexuality has been affected by pregnancy and parenting. Check out "Sex and Parenting," a section devoted to the sexuality of parents and kids, written by Anne and sponsored by Good Vibrations.

Jewish Family and Life

http://www.jewishfamily.com/features/996/talking.htm

You know what the experts say, but you're wondering how to frame your sex talk in the context of your religious beliefs? Visit Jewish Family and Life for valuable communication tips and suggestions (relevant to all faiths) for reconciling conflicting family values.

Parents, Friends and Families of Lesbians and Gays (PFLAG)

http://www.pflag.org

We all want to be loved for who we are, and this organization exists so that families and friends of gays and lesbians can show the world the meaning of unconditional love and acceptance. PFLAG has over 70,000 members who voice this message loud and clear and are active in community organizing; the press releases posted on the site will keep you abreast of the latest challenges to gay rights. You can click on a map of the United States to find contact information for whichever one of PFLAG's four hundred chapters is nearest you. The organization sells several publications aimed at helping families support their gay children, and the site features tips on working with gay youth aimed at teachers, counselors, and health professionals. PFLAG posts a monthly question that visitors to the site are invited to answer. All responses are posted the following month and serve as an enlightening and poignant reflection on gay and family life in America. Our only suggestion is that the questions be archived by topic rather than by date, so they are easier to view.

ParentTime

http://www.pathfinder.com/ParentTime

It's late, you've chewed your nails down to the quick, and your daughter still hasn't come home from her date. Need someone to talk to? Log on to one of the chat rooms at ParentTime and share your anxiety with other parents burning the midnight oil. This site also offers discussion boards on various topics and transcripts of past chats, so you can view previous discussions on relevant subjects. Dr. Ruth also contributes a sex advice column for kids and parents. Elsewhere on this site Michele Bitoun Blecher's *Parenting* magazine article teaches you how to tailor your "birds and bees" talk to a child's specific mental disability. She stresses the role of repetition and the importance of supporting your child's exploration.

Planned Parenthood National Site

http://www.plannedparenthood.org

In your lifetime you will make countless decisions that affect your sexual health—from choosing birth control to choosing partners, from planning your own sex education to planning your child's. You would be hard-pressed to find a better resource to help you make well-informed, intelligent decisions along the way than Planned Parenthood. Their voluminous Web site houses much of the literature they've distributed through their clinics, written in language designed to be thorough, clear, and accessible to adults of various educational levels—one of the main reasons Planned Parenthood's program is so effective.

Planned Parenthood is well known for its support of reproductive freedoms, but the public is less aware of the organization's rigorous commitment to sex education. Alongside the information on contraception, pregnancy, and abortion, you'll discover a vast array of articles for parents and teachers about how to raise sexually healthy kids. For example, did you know that by the age of five, children should be familiar with the correct names for their genitals, feel comfortable asking a trusted adult questions about sexuality, and be able to talk about body parts without a sense of "naughtiness"? For guidelines outlining age-appropriate sex information, check out the article entitled "Human Sexuality: What Children Should Know and When They Should Know It." These guidelines are especially useful for anyone who's ever said, "My child is not old enough to know that yet!"

The site also includes short sections about puberty, anatomy (with illustrations), menstruation, and making decisions about sex. The site is extremely well organized, with ample cross-referencing and a search feature to help you zero in on the desired information.

Precocious Puberty General Information

http://www.cmhcsys.com/factsfam/puberty.htm

Parents of children experiencing "precocious puberty"—the premature onset of puberty, which affects one in ten thousand children—can get help from the Precocious Puberty General Information site. By discovering what emotional, behavioral, and physiological changes to expect, you can explore ways to treat and ease this difficult period in your child's life.

Resources for Parents of Gay, Lesbian, Bi and Transgendered Youth

http://www.pe.net/~bidstrup/parents.htm

Authored by Scott Bidstrup, a self-described "secular humanist liberal gay cowboy" (and former Mormon) whose personal passion is helping dispossessed gay youth, this site is designed both to reassure parents whose kids have come out and to offer information and tools for supporting their gay, lesbian, bisexual, or transgendered children. The site includes answers to common medical, legal, religious, and cultural questions raised by a child's coming out; tips on providing your child with support within his or her community and school system; and links to other resources, including the homepages of individual activists and PFLAG (Parents, Friends and Families of Lesbians and Gays). Scott also hosts the "Cool Page for Queer Teens," providing similar reassurance and resources for kids.

Sexuality Information and Education Council of the United States (SIECUS)

http://www.siecus.org

Founded on the belief that sexuality is a natural and healthy part of living, SIECUS is a national nonprofit that advocates for the individual's right to make responsible sexual choices. To that end, SIECUS researches and distributes accurate sex information, particularly throughout elementary and high schools. This site is most useful to teachers and parents who want to learn about or develop a comprehensive sex education program for children. Its somewhat scholarly focus will discourage casual readers, but those who persist will be rewarded with thought-provoking analyses of everything from "Media Recommendations for More Realistic, Accurate Images Concerning Sexuality" and "Religious Right and Fear Based Sex Education" to "Condom Effectiveness and Use" and "Life Behaviors of a Sexually Healthy Adult."

SIECUS has developed an excellent set of resources, pamphlets, and exercises to help adults speak comfortably and knowledgeably with kids about sex (particularly, the pamphlet "Now What Do I Do?"). Anyone looking for further reading material will appreciate the annotated bibliographies on dozens of subjects, including general sexuality, adolescent sexuality, sex and disability, religious perspectives, teaching materials, sexual orientation, sex and pop culture, and child sexual abuse. Unfortunately, this site suffers from a repetitive, unimaginative layout that can be confusing. It's not always easy to tell where you are, what's for sale and how to order it, and what's been excerpted from longer articles.

Talking to Your Children About AIDS: Mother's Voices

http://mvoices.org/talk.htm

For mind-blowing statistics that will convince you that it's important to talk to kids about safer sex, visit Talking to Your Children About AIDS: Mother's Voices. For example, a study of mothers and their adolescent children found that 70 percent of the mothers believed their sons were virgins, but only 44 percent of those sons actually were. You'll learn more about *why* you should talk to your kids than *how*, but you'll also find some great resources, a discussion board, and suggestions for how to involve your kids' schools in sex education.

Texas' Planned Parenthood

http://www.pphouston.org

Pull two chairs up to your computer and engage in a little hands-on dialogue with your child, courtesy of Texas' Planned Parenthood activity pages. Kids can interview their parents about body image and other issues that concerned them when they were young, and teens can swap lists with parents about messages they were given about sex.

KIDS

All About Sex

http://www.allaboutsex.org

This site gets an A for intent, a B for follow-through, and a C for presentation. We commend its webmaster for creating a site where parents and children are invited to come share their thoughts about sex: "The primary goal of this project is to get people to open their minds to ideas about sex that our society in the past has not been able to discuss openly and rationally." To that end, he establishes separate discussion forums for parents, preteens, and teens and poses age-appropriate, thought-provoking questions to each audience. Preteens can discuss masturbation, teens can talk about sexual orientation or deciding when to have sex, and adults can swap ideas about sexual politics. So far, there's not a lot of activity within the forums, for a few reasons: the site is in its infancy and large portions are still under construction; posting feedback is somewhat cumbersome; and the author's opinions, though well intended, can be long-winded and preachy. Unfortunately, the site's design—multiple colors of reverse type, small fonts, and a background galaxy pattern with pulsating planets—discourages lingering on any page too long and is bound to deter reader participation. However, there's a welcome humor section, as well as an illuminating tribute to a variety of sexual pioneers, and we're optimistic that this promising site will mature into an essential destination on your child's sex education tour.

Coalition for Positive Sexuality

http://www.positive.org

"You have the right to make your own choices, and to have people respect them." That message to teens from the coalition—a group of high-school students and adults dedicated to educating teens about sex—comes through loud and clear on their Web site. The coalition's primary goal is to give teens vital sex information and to affirm their decisions about sex, sexuality, and reproductive control. Its secondary goal is to get sex education and condom distribution programs into high schools.

In response to the political and media campaign admonishing kids to "just say no," CPS authored a booklet called *Just Say Yes*, which appears online in its entirety, in both English and Spanish. It covers a variety of sexual issues—including sexual self-esteem, respect, consent, sexual orientation, safer sex, sex toys, communication, STDs, pregnancy, and abortion. Its colorful, streetwise language should be particularly appealing to teens. The site also features a FAQ section, a chat room populated by dozens of sex-positive teens, and good links. Staff members answer submitted questions privately, and a search function allows users to find the information they seek quickly. Nice presentation and extremely easy to navigate.

Doctor Paula's Site

http://www.drpaula.com

Pediatrician Paula Elbirt's site offers a section in which teens can learn about sexuality, orgasm, masturbation, sexual pressure, talking with parents, contraception, body changes, and erections. The information is sound and the essays brief, which is entirely appropriate for younger readers. She offers eleven basic tips for parents on how to talk with kids about sex. For example, you may already know that it's unwise to laugh at or ignore your child's sex questions, but are you also looking for teachable moments, praising his or her questions (thereby reinforcing that you are approachable), and trying not to

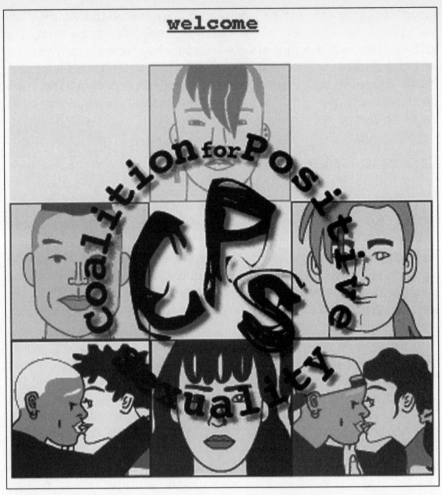

welcome

Copyright©Coalition for Positive Sexuality Web design: Brad Borevitz, Push It Web Development

overestimate your child's knowledge? The sex information is a bit buried within the site, but a search function alleviates this problem somewhat.

Elight

http://www.elight.org

Most parents never bother to discuss sexual orientation with kids, which is one reason online resources can be especially useful to the gay teen. Written by and for queer youth, the zine *Elight* features dozens of touching coming-out stories submitted by readers and a bulletin board for "ranting and raving" about gay life.

Go Ask Alice!

http://www.goaskalice.columbia.edu

If you've ever wished for a sex version of "Dear Abby," you're ready for Go Ask Alice! Maintained by Columbia University's Health Services Department, this site receives hundreds of questions each week on every conceivable aspect of sexuality. Thank heavens for the search function! See p. 104 for a longer review.

Kotex Girl Space and Tampax's Troom

http://www.kotex.com/girlspace and http://www.troom.com

When the cat's got your tongue and you need a little help explaining menstruation and puberty to your daughter, send her to Kotex Girl Space or Tampax's Troom. Sure, they explain the how-tos of their products, but these sites are also a gold mine of information and reassurance. She'll get help charting her cycle, advice about cramps, answers to popular questions about puberty, exercises to help with self-esteem, and the opportunity to sound off with other girls in a discussion board. (A tip: parents who lurk in a discussion board room can learn a lot about what their kids are going through.)

Puberty in Boys

http://www.public.health.wa.gov.au/hp2106.htm

This informative site, sponsored by the Health Department of Western Australia, is designed to reassure adolescent boys about the emotional and physical changes running rampant in their lives. Delivered in a straightforward, nonjudgmental style, the site offers basic facts about puberty, covering everything from acne, wet dreams, and penis size to masturbation, relationships, and sexual health. The discussion of genital anatomy would benefit from a few illustrations, but overall the site is both helpful and accessible.

Safer Sex Pages

http://www.safersex.org

Whatever your preference or question, the Safer Sex Pages can help you. Parents who aren't entirely comfortable demonstrating condom use to their children might choose to view the video clip of a condom slipping over a dildo. Kids might choose the illustrated cartoons. The lesbian unsure of what constitutes unsafe sex between women might print the site's cutout guidelines to display next to her bed. The information and language are geared toward teens, but most adults will improve their own safer-sex knowledge with a visit to this page. See p. 99 for a longer review.

Web by Women for Women and English Server

http://www.io.com/~wwwomen/sexuality/ready
http://eserver.org/feminism/guide-to-condoms.txt

A young woman considering sex for the first time could not find a better sounding board than the Web by Women for Women's "First Time" section. The site's thought-provoking advice and firsthand accounts will steer her toward making an informed, responsible decision and give her all the helpful information she needs on contraception and safer sex. When the time comes to whip out her first condom, she'll know how to put it on correctly after reading "A Girl's Guide to Condoms," located on the English Server site (see p. 87).

Chapter Six

SHOPPING

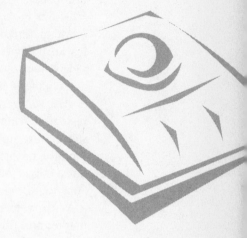

Let Your Modem Do the Shopping

Have you ever purchased an "adult" product in person? If so, you probably had to grapple with a few anxieties that don't surface during your average trip to the grocery store. Maybe you were worried that someone you know—say a fellow member of the PTA, your mom, or a co-worker—would spot you entering the store, that the sales clerk would snicker at your question about butt plugs, or that the person waiting behind you in line would raise her eyebrows at the porn video you shyly placed on the counter. It's not easy to conquer your fears and cross the threshold of a sex store—and even if you're willing to give it a shot, you may not live in a community where there are places to shop for sexual materials.

Thanks to the Web, you can say good-bye to anxiety and hello to total access. Now you can browse the virtual shelves of a limitless variety of erotic emporiums without ever leaving the privacy of your own home. You can make purchases at any hour of the day or night, ask questions via e-mail without embarrassment, and glean sex information with a simple click of the mouse. With Internet sales expected to exceed mail-order catalog sales within a few years, it should come as no surprise that a substantial share of the billions generated by online commerce will be from sales of sexual products.

After all, the Web's irresistible combination of discretion, accessibility, and convenience is tailor-made for sex shopping, and sex shopping itself is on the rise throughout the country. According to a 1997 National Sexual Health Survey, 10 percent of sexually active adults—nearly fourteen million people—report using sex toys, alone and with their partners. And the 1994 *Sex in America* survey found that up to 20 percent of adults purchase erotic materials in any given year. Mainstream publishers are releasing erotica anthologies by the dozens, and the rise in female consumers of adult videos—an estimated 40 percent of all adult video rentals are to women and couples—is gradually revitalizing the X-rated video industry.

Are you getting the picture? Sexual products are big business. So the next time you're sitting in a boring meeting or lecture, entertain yourself by speculating how many people in the room keep a Hitachi Magic Wand vibrator plugged in by the bed, spent the previous evening watching the latest Vivid Video release, or just purchased this year's edition of *Best American Erotica*. Sex consumers are everywhere!

With women comprising an ever-growing segment of both the online market and the market for sexual products, numerous "cyberboutiques" are following the model that has made women-friendly retail outlets so successful offline: they woo increasingly savvy consumers with quality products, comprehensive services, accurate information, and a philosophical attitude that inspires trust. Many of our survey respondents emphasized that they base their shopping decisions on company identity. As one woman comments, "I don't want to shop from a 'Sleaze! Dirt! Wickedness! Naked Hot Mamas' site. The only site I'd be interested in looking around, let alone buying from, would be one that gave the impression it was run by and catered to intelligent adults of both genders who think sex is a fun and healthy way to get some pleasure out of life."

Even businesses that have not traditionally catered to women are taking notice of their presence online. The Adam & Eve print catalog mails to a list that is made up of about 80 percent men, and adult videos are its number-one seller. Yet one-third of the orders from the online Adam & Eve catalog are to women, and vibrators are the biggest sellers online. As these kind of demographic shifts take place, there's bound to be an accompanying shift in content and presentation geared toward female consumers.

The world of online shopping is actually ideally suited to showcase a company's attitude and philosophy. Web sites offer the luxury of limitless pages in which to present detailed product, company, and sex information, unlike retail stores and catalogs, which are constrained by the cost of floor space, paper, and postage. Online, it's not unusual to find sexpert advice,

CONCERNS ABOUT ONLINE ORDERING

Web surfers responding to a survey conducted by the Better Business Bureau cited fear of credit card fraud as the number-one reason for choosing not to order online. In fact, online fraud is of the same garden variety that exists offline—the kind that puts your credit card at risk when it leaves your hands, even briefly, in day-to-day use. While a customer service representative could steal your card number from your order, or your next-door neighbor could pilfer your receipts out of the trash and go on a shopping spree, these possibilities probably haven't stopped you from shopping before, and there's no reason they should now. Furthermore, most credit card companies have a policy of covering fraudulent charges of over fifty dollars (which is actually a good reason to pay by credit card if you're nervous about a company's legitimacy).

Fear of Internet fraud gets fueled by images of joyriding hackers waiting to intercept credit card numbers as they're transmitted over the Internet, despite the fact that there have been no reported cases of this (perhaps because the hackers are too busy cracking Department of Defense files). Nonetheless, to reduce the risk, many companies implement "secure" online ordering software.

Secure Sockets Layer (SSL) and Secure Hypertext Transfer Protocol (SHTTP) are standard industry protocols; these programs encrypt your personal information as it travels over the Internet, making your name, address, and credit card number all but impossible to unscramble. When you are about to submit your order, it's easy to check whether you're in a secure environment by looking at the bottom of your browser. It will either show a gold key, which should be solid, not broken, or a padlock, which should appear locked.

We also advise you to relax! Some smaller online companies don't have secure ordering capabilities. In many cases, they will suggest alternative precautions, such as sending each half of your credit card number in two different e-mails, or sending your credit card number in a combination of numbers and words. We would hate to see mom-and-pop (or mom-and-mom and pop-and-pop) businesses penalized for not being able to afford the latest technology. Consider adopting their suggested strategies, or if you'd rather not use your credit card online—or you don't have one—you can almost always place your order via phone, fax, or mail.

columns on everything from G-spot stimulation to negotiating an S/M scene, interviews with adult stars, sex FAQs, excerpts from books, or clips from videos accompanying the merchandise for sale. You can learn how a company was founded and who's behind it, as well as enjoy links to related companies.

Furthermore, the Web offers an edge over retail stores and mail-order catalogs when it comes to comparison shopping. In person, you probably wouldn't have the option of traveling to five or six different sex toy stores in order to locate the best price or selection. And though mail order offers convenience and privacy, few people welcome the prospect of adult catalogs flooding their mailboxes (and few would ever go to the trouble of systematically comparing and contrasting different catalogs). On the Web, you can visit a dozen stores within an hour, and the time you spend shopping around will almost always be rewarded in savings. Even better, the heavy competition and low costs of online cataloging are likely to keep online prices down for the foreseeable future. An added bonus is the online convention of using incentives to coax shoppers to a new medium: many more cyberstores offer free gifts, discounts, and monthly prizes than do offline stores or mail-order catalogs.

What's more, as online software becomes more refined, the Web promises to elevate customer service to new heights. Based on your previous visits, online shops will be able to route you information that's specifically tailored to your preferences or interests. This may be the closest thing

---

SHOPPING TIPS

So you've decided to sample some of the exotic wares available online—what's next? There are plenty of wonderful companies waiting to make all your retail dreams come true—like the ones mentioned here—but there are also those lying in wait to scam a quick buck. Your best strategy is to be prepared, so here are a few guidelines to ensure a happy shopping excursion.

Finding a Company You Like

Go with what you know. It may sound obvious, but if you already trust and patronize a particular adult store or mail-order company, look for its Web site.

Rely on name recognition. If you remember reading favorable comments about certain companies in a newspaper or magazine, or if you've seen their advertising in reputable publications, chances are good that they're not fly-by-night operations.

Get recommendations from friends. Friends who share your tastes can be an excellent source of leads. If you participate in any online discussion groups, ask for referrals.

Use links from your favorite sex information sites. In other words, if you trust a site, trust its links. Links can be as helpful as personal

referrals in helping you zero in on specialized resources. For example, S/M sites will refer you to manufacturers of bondage gear, and safer-sex sites will refer you to condom shops.

Look for a mission statement. To distinguish themselves from the masses of carbon-copy adult sites, many companies post a personal or mission statement, which gives you a sense of who's behind the site.

Don't put too much stock in awards. Anyone can create and distribute Web site awards, so there's no point in being impressed by such plaudits (unless they're bestowed by a well-known outfit such as Yahoo!). Awards tend to be gimmicks designed to trick you into visiting the award-giver's site; some are based on the number of hits a site receives, which doesn't reflect the site's quality as much as its marketing savvy.

Don't judge a book by its cover. Large adult companies can afford to pay for graphic design, while cottage businesses often rely on a do-it-yourself approach. What smaller or offbeat sites lack in elegant design, they may well make up for in personality and customer service. As one of our survey respondents noted, it's more important that a site be "nicely made with a feel of love!"

you'll ever get to a personal sex toy shopper! Some people are skittish about what they perceive to be the Big Brother implications of having their surfing pattern and their purchasing history tracked with "cookies" (the term for the bits of data stored on your computer as you browse through a Web site). If you choose, you can set your browser to notify you when a cookie is on your trail and refuse it. However, once you've found a vendor you trust, you'll probably come to appreciate customized messages letting you know that your favorite brand of lube is on sale, or that Pat Califia's new book has just been released.

Despite these advantages, many consumers still have reservations about shopping online. By far the most common concern expressed is fear of credit

Verify a company's legitimacy. A toll-free number is a good (but not foolproof) indication that a company is at least established enough to foot the bill for your call. Order copies of any catalogs or brochures before placing an online order, or if the company doesn't offer any print materials, ask for additional references. If you're really dubious about a particular company, check with the Better Business Bureau or Internet Fraud Watch to see if any complaints have been filed against it (see "Consumer Resources," p. 77). After all this, if you're still suspicious, shop elsewhere.

Check the company's confidentiality policy. Many adult companies promise not to sell or rent your street or e-mail address to other companies, but don't assume this is the case. Check their stated policy, and while you're at it, ask how discreet their packaging is.

Placing an Order

Look for specific products by description, not by name. Adult retailers often make up their own names for toys, so even if all your friends are raving about the Jelly G-Spot Vibrator or the King Kong Dildo, don't restrict yourself to searching for it by this name. If you have a physical description, you improve your chances of locating the toy at the best price.

Research customer service policies before you place your order. What is the company's return policy on unwanted or defective items? When can you expect to receive your order? If this information isn't clearly posted on the site, e-mail the company for an answer. Any mail-order company is legally obligated to deliver your order within thirty days, unless you have approved a longer period (for instance, on a back-ordered item). If a company can't deliver within this time frame, you are entitled to a full refund.

Pay attention to shipping charges. You may find a good price on a product only to see the savings eaten up by excessive freight charges. Or you might prefer to buy your condoms for $2.50 at the drug store rather than fork over $5.00 in shipping. In any case, it's worth shopping around for competitive shipping rates.

Choose the ordering method you're most comfortable with. For more information, see the sidebar "Concerns About Online Ordering" (p. 127).

Always print out a copy of the order. This will come in handy should you need to file a complaint.

If you're not satisfied, complain. For tips on how to get restitution, see "If You Get Ripped Off" (p. 64).

card theft or fraud, to which we can only respond—have you been shopping offline lately?! In reality, it's no more risky to transmit your credit card number over the Internet than over the phone—and it's probably less risky than handing over your card in a crowded store or busy restaurant. Sure, it's possible for someone to hack into a company's files during transmission and steal your card, but this is extremely unlikely. You can further reduce this minimal risk by shopping from companies with secure online ordering capabilities (see our "Concerns About Online Ordering" sidebar, p. 127, for details). And if you're still uneasy at the prospect of your credit card number traveling over the wires, you can research your purchase online and place your actual order the old-fashioned way: by phone, fax, or mail.

Of course, plenty of shoppers feel there's no substitute for actually handling a product before they make a purchase. While this is true, online catalogs can offer a uniquely thorough introduction to products. The tiny photos or drawings in a mail-order catalog can't compare with the detailed presentations of merchandise you can find on a Web site. And a sales clerk working in a crowded or understaffed store can't necessarily provide the comprehensive tips on product selection that you can glean from a Web site.

Overall, consumers of adult products emerge as winners in the shift to online shopping. The Web offers not only unprecedented access to sex information but high standards of responsiveness and accountability—word travels fast through online communities. For years, adult businesses have exploited sexual ignorance and embarrassment in order to get away with offering inferior products at exorbitant prices. The Web is the ideal environment in which to nurture a new breed of savvy, discriminating, and demanding adult consumers who won't settle for less. While sexual embarrassment isn't likely to vanish with the wave of a Hitachi Magic Wand, at least the Web allows you to shop around and compare notes with other consumers in total anonymity—and to educate yourself in the process. However, with literally hundreds of sex shops on the Web, narrowing the field to those that suit your tastes can be a daunting and time-consuming task. To help get you started, we've reviewed a variety of reputable businesses that sell a wide range of toys, books, and videos.

A Sex Shop of Her Own

Over the past twenty-five years, the proprietors of women-run sex shops have revolutionized adult retailing. By taking a "clean, well-lighted" approach to the merchandising of sexual products, they have normalized the pursuit of sexual pleasure for women and men alike. Pioneering stores such as New York's Eve's Garden and San Francisco's Good Vibrations arose out of the consciousness-raising and feminist self-help movements of the '70s. Dell Williams was inspired by the teachings of Wilhelm Reich, her experience coordinating NOW's first women's sexuality conference, and her friendship with Betty Dodson—the erotic artist behind the famed women's Bodysex masturbation workshops—to open Eve's Garden in 1974. Joani Blank, a sex therapist and educator with a degree in public health, opened Good Vibrations in 1977 after the women in her preorgasmic women's groups complained that there was nowhere they felt comfortable shopping for vibrators. Both these women started out with the goal of creating a friendly, nonthreatening environment in which women could access sexual information and products, but of course, the sex-positive atmosphere of their stores was irresistible to many men as well.

Women-run sex stores set out to distinguish themselves from run-of-the-mill adult bookstores in ambiance, presentation, and selection. In contrast to adult bookstores—where most products are shrink-wrapped and hung on the wall or placed behind a counter—stores such as Good Vibrations displayed samples of every product, so that customers could test each vibrator's buzz, touch and taste lubricants, or browse through books. Staff people were trained to answer questions about sexual anatomy and response and to let customers know both the advantages and the drawbacks of every product sold. These stores functioned as community clearinghouses—advice, information, referrals, and reassurance flowed like lube at a sex party.

Above all, these stores developed an exceptional selection of toys, bringing together items that had never before been available under one roof: brand-name massagers (useful for so much more than back massages), novelty vibrators, and a treasure trove of products from creative entrepreneurs. Yes, we have America's women-run sex stores to thank for nurturing technological innovations such as the silicone dildo, the leather dildo harness, and the rainbow-colored array of battery vibrators that today's consumers take for granted! Mainstream adult manufacturers, who focused on importing the same old cheesy novelties and selling them at ludicrous markups through established distribution channels, had no interest in catering to a "boutique" market or in working on a better mousetrap. But the consumer-friendly atmosphere of the women's stores created a more educated clientele, and cottage industries sprang up in response to the growing demand for quality goods.

Once the women's stores proved that there is a substantial market for higher-priced, well-made toys, mainstream manufacturers began to put some energy into improving the quality and design of their own products. However, the boutique stores remain the most reliable source for specialty items that you won't find in an adult bookstore. In selecting which stores to review, we were admittedly biased in favor of those that showcase the work of creative sexual entrepreneurs. After all, you can find a battery-operated

"I have learned a lot about self-pleasure, as well as the pleasure and sensuality of using adult toys with a partner."

vibrating egg in a thousand different places, but to find a Vixen dildo, a Wondrous Vulva hand puppet, or a Betty Dodson video for sale, you'll need to patronize some pretty select outfits!

It should come as no surprise that the owners of women's sex stores were quick to recognize the Web's potential for networking on a global scale. Virtual versions of these welcoming, community-oriented storefronts are appearing all over cyberspace. As Good Vibrations's webmistress Krissy Cababa explains, "We put up a site to further our mission of dispensing accurate information about sex to as wide an audience as possible." And Ellen Barnard of A Woman's Touch points out, "Having a site means we are achieving one of our biggest goals: to provide helpful information about relationships and sexuality in an environment that is comfortable and safe for both women and men. It never fails to touch me that we get e-mail at least once a day thanking us for having the site, and telling us how much the site has made a difference in someone's life."

The beauty of the Web is that, through their educational endeavors, these small businesses can have an effect quite disproportionate to their size. The site for A Woman's Touch features regularly updated advice columns on health and relationships, and Ellen notes that as a result, search engines point browsers to their site "with words as diverse as *sex, vibrators, orgasms, impotence, restraints*, and *nipples.*" Sex information sites all over the country link to Good Vibrations's posted "Ten Rules of Anal Sex" and "About the G-Spot," while owner Kim Airs is awed that her Grand Opening! site generates orders from as far away as Africa and Asia. Within a year or two of establishing their sites, many of these businesses find that the Web accounts for 10 to 25 percent of their total sales and brings visitors to their stores who previously had never known they existed.

The Web also provides an opportunity to combine commerce with entertainment—to deliver the message that sex can be both fun and funny. An article stating that sex toys have been around throughout human history may be edifying, but it's probably less memorable than a tour of the Good Vibrations Antique Vibrator Museum, in which photos of vintage vibrators are paired with commentary suggesting, for example, how Queen Victoria might have cheered herself up after the demise of her beloved Albert. And anyone who's seen the photo of Kim Airs dressed up as the Grand Opening! logo—a gift-wrapped box—is unlikely to fear being intimidated by shopping at her store.

The warmth and personality of many of these innovative, pioneering women comes through loud and clear in their sites. We can't think of a more appropriate way to send you off on your tour of the best women's sex stores than with Ellen Barnard's explanation of how she decided to open A Woman's Touch: "A couple of years ago while I was trying to decide what I wanted to do next in life, I realized that the Midwest didn't have a comfortable place for women to celebrate and explore our sexuality. Upon telling my grandmother this, she replied 'Well, get working on it, because I can't wait to tell my friends that my granddaughter runs a sex store!' Although my grandmother died a week before we opened, she always believed in me and was proud of what I was doing, so this store is for grandma, and all the great, feisty women like her."

Reviews

A few general characteristics apply to all the companies that follow, so we have noted only exceptions to the rules in our reviews. Unless noted, all update their sites monthly, weekly, or daily—with monthly updates being most common. By and large, prices—particularly in the women-owned stores—are comparable. Return policies for "intimate products" tend to be much less generous than those for other consumer goods (after all, you can't open an outlet store for reject dildos). Many adult companies accept returns only on unused items, and—because of the ease of duplication—most won't accept returns on videos. Those with liberal return policies often compensate by setting slightly higher prices for their products. We've noted which companies have satisfaction guarantees on their entire product line, but even those with less generous return policies frequently bend the rules for the sake of keeping customers happy.

Since confidentiality is such a concern for consumers of sexual materials, most reputable adult businesses have a policy of not selling, renting, or trading their customers' names. Unless noted, all the companies we review here have a stated policy guaranteeing confidentiality, so there's no way you're going to find yourself on a "smut-lovers" mailing list.

Finally, we've indicated which companies also offer a print catalog.

WOMEN-RUN BUSINESSES

Eve's Garden

http://www.evesgarden.com

The online version of the first feminist sex store in the country is well worth a visit simply to check out founder Dell Williams's thoughtful responses to frequently asked questions about vibrators. A Wilhelm Reich enthusiast, Dell exhorts us that "Sexual energy is the fire that warms our heart, kindles our creativity, and lights our spirit. Come Celebrate the Joy." We particularly appreciate her response to the age-old question, Why do I need a vibrator? "You don't need it. You choose it. And if you do, it is a wonderful way to learn about your own sexual response, your own body, your own orgasms. Using a vibrator is a personal journey into self pleasuring . . . a celebration of your own sexuality. Loving yourself is a first step toward shared love."

The product selection includes a full range of toys and self-help books, and a limited selection of educational and erotic videos. Eve's Garden is an attractive site, but you may want to simply check out what's available and then order a free print catalog online, since responsiveness to the site—which is infrequently updated—can be slow. Or if you're in New York City, visit the store itself.

Good Vibrations

http://www.goodvibes.com

"Promoting sexual health and pleasure since 1977," this women-owned, worker-owned business comprises two retail stores in the San Francisco Bay Area, The Sexuality Library and the Good Vibrations mail-order catalogs, and Down There Press, a publisher of sex-related books. Good Vibrations brings to cyberspace a unique blend of down-to-earth information, sex trivia, entertainment, thoughtfully selected merchandise, and missionary zeal. We both worked at Good Vibes for over ten years, so we can't pretend to be objective, but—trust us!—no trip online is complete without a visit to this site.

Step right up to see the world-renowned Antique Vibrator Museum: photographs of vibrators that date back to the turn of the century, accompanied by theories about which famous people throughout history could (or should) have used them. Monthly columns by Carol Queen and Pat Califia, answers to sex questions submitted by customers, comprehensive tips on how to select and care for your toy, product recommendations from fellow customers, and the "Did You Know?" column of sex trivia will all boost your sexual literacy. And of course, there are toys, books, and videos galore—the selection of erotic and educational books and videos is particularly strong. The site is simple and easy to navigate. Products are presented with colorful line drawings and friendly blurbs and are cross-referenced with informational tidbits about anatomy, sexual

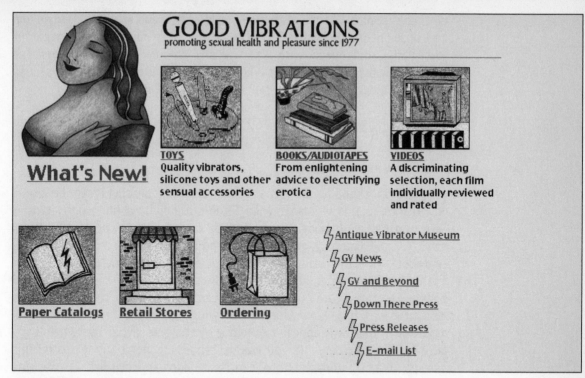

GOOD VIBRATIONS
promoting sexual health and pleasure since 1977

What's New!

TOYS
Quality vibrators, silicone toys and other sensual accessories

BOOKS/AUDIOTAPES
From enlightening advice to electrifying erotica

VIDEOS
A discriminating selection, each film individually reviewed and rated

Paper Catalogs **Retail Stores** **Ordering**

Antique Vibrator Museum
GV News
GV and Beyond
Down There Press
Press Releases
E-mail List

response, and how to select the right toy for you. Online ordering is secure, and you can request free print catalogs either online or by calling a toll-free number.

Grand Opening! Sexuality Boutique

http://www.grandopening.com

Grand Opening! (yup, the exclamation mark is part of the name) is a Boston store founded in 1993 "to provide women and men with a comfortable place to shop for items to enhance their sexuality." The company's most valuable asset is its warm and wacky owner, Kim Airs. Kim's enthusiastic, encouraging personality comes through loud and clear in her cozy little online boutique.

Visit Grand Opening! and you can enjoy a slide show of Kim posed in front of different product groupings or dressed up as the store's logo (a gift-wrapped package); find out if Kim's coming to your town to lead a workshop (on topics from female ejaculation to developing a "drag king" persona); get linked to other women-friendly businesses and women sex pioneers; and most important, go shopping. The mood throughout is friendly and inclusive; women and men of all orientations will feel welcome at this site. Grand Opening! offers sex toys, books, and videos, with a particularly thorough selection of toys. The site's simple presentation makes it easy to navigate. Online ordering is secure, or you can order from a toll-free number. Updates are infrequent.

In Harmony

http://www.in-harmony.com

One-stop shopping for sensuous and sexual products can be yours thanks to this woman-owned Texas outfit, whose philosophy is that "every part of your body deserves to be cared for in loving and healthful ways . . . that you may know pleasure and harmony." The merchandise presentation—of bath, skin care, and aromatherapy products, a couple of leather items, vibrators, lubricants, jewelry, and a few sex-related videos and books—is utterly bare-bones. Products are listed simply by category and illustrated with black-and-white line drawings. However, this is a thoughtful assortment that will appeal to anyone wishing to avoid overwhelmingly large product selections. (If you wonder why there aren't any dildos on this site, you might be interested to learn that dildos are classified as "obscene devices" in the state of Texas, where their sale is technically illegal.) The reasonable prices and sex-positive attitude are another draw. Online ordering is secure, and a print catalog is available for a fee.

Nice -N- Naughty

http://www.nice-n-naughty.com

Katherine, the charming proprietress of this site, is a former home-party sex toy saleswoman who discovered the wider online community while a member of CompuServe's Human Sexuality and Relationships Forum. Her online shop is somewhat confusing in presentation—you select from a grid of product categories set against a backdrop of stars—and overwhelming (do we really need Yanni music playing while we shop?), but Katherine's warm presence and sensible advice are capable of redeeming even the eye-straining reverse type.

The assortment of toys, books, and videos is thorough, and each product category is introduced with tips on how to select and enjoy your toys. Katherine scrupulously reminds potential customers that individual tastes and responses will vary, frankly explains the drawbacks of the adult industry, and passes on customer feedback from her devoted clientele of women and men. She also lists the addresses and toll-free numbers of organizations and hotlines dealing with abuse, AIDS, rape, sexuality, and BDSM. Check out her enthusiastic vibrator introduction, with advice ranging from the philosophical (love me, love my vibrator) to the practical (leave paper in the vibrator's battery compartment to reduce noise). Online ordering is secure, or you can order using Nice -N- Naughty's toll-free number.

Toys in Babeland

http://www.babeland.com

The friendly, personable gals behind Seattle's Toys in Babeland claim they "sell sex toys to make money, make friends, and change the world." This good-humored attitude is evident throughout their site. Products are presented with simple line drawings and informative descriptions. As you'd expect, Toys in Babeland is particularly well stocked with toys, but the site also has a good, select assortment of books and videos for women. Extra benefits of this "S/M, transgender, queer, straight, vanilla, and bi friendly" site include installments from *Girlfriends* magazine's "Girltoy" column—an excellent blend of product reviews and testimonials penned by one of Toys in Babeland's owners. The site's lesbian e-zine, *Squeezebox*, and advice column, "Talk is Cheap," are equally entertaining, if infrequently updated—as is the entire site. Online ordering is secure, and you can request a free print catalog either online or by calling a toll-free number.

Vixen Creations

http://www.tenderbuttons.com/vixen

Vixen Creations, a small manufacturer based in San Francisco, designs and produces the most innovative, elegant silicone dildos in the country. These dildos literally inspire rhapsodies from appreciative customers, who no doubt agree with Vixen's motto, "Worth every inch." They're made of a sleek, silky silicone that is miraculously resistant to breaking and available in a range of rich, jewel-toned hues (including glitter and glow-in-the-dark) that look good enough to eat. The Vixen site doesn't accept orders, but it does offer the opportunity to survey the entire line; each dildo is featured in its own large cameo-style photo. Links to all the companies that carry Vixen products serve as a useful guide to women-owned and women-friendly shops around the country. One link will lead you to "The Packy Page," devoted to a Vixen product designed especially for female-to-male transsexuals.

A Woman's Touch

http://www.a-womans-touch.com

The online version of this Madison, Wisconsin, store is an exceptionally interactive site with much to offer surfers interested in "sensuality and sexual pleasure from women's perspectives." Owners Myrtle and Ellen, formerly employed as a doctor and a social worker, are as dedicated to providing sex information and encouragement as they are to selling products. As Myrtle notes, "unlike Joycelyn Elders, M.D., I can keep my job as long as I talk to the public about masturbation . . . what a deal."

The site's "Ask Dr. Myrtle" advice column is an excellent source of information on sexuality, as well as sexual and reproductive health, covering topics from STDs to hormonal changes to sex toys. The "Ask Aphrodite" column offers love and relationship advice. Both columns are updated regularly. The product line encompasses toys, books, videos, and select items of lingerie (including large sizes); thorough descriptions accompany all items, and online ordering is secure.

Womyns' Ware

http://www.womynsware.com

Womyns' Ware is a Canadian store and mail-order catalog owned by two "lesbian witches" dedicated to celebrating and empowering women's sexuality. They provide an excellent cross-section of toys (including some exclusive items) and a handful of self-help books. The layout is a little frame-happy, which limits the size of the screen containing product information, but you don't need much room to get the effect of the simple line drawings and accompanying blurbs, and it's easy to find your way around the site. Prices are listed in Canadian and U.S. dollars. There is no online ordering, except through e-mail, but a toll-free number is provided. The service-oriented approach of the store's owners is reflected in their regular newsletter and their "Fucking Good" sex advice column, which appears in *LezzieSmut* magazine—both are posted on the site.

Adam & Eve

http://www.adameve.com

America's largest adult catalog company—with over four million customers to date—presents an online "garden of earthly delights." You'll find a basic array of low-end sex toys (no electric vibrators or silicone dildos here), videos galore, lingerie, and a sampling of books. Adam & Eve's presentation is admittedly cheesy (think porn starlets peeling bananas), and their target customers clearly are men, but there's plenty for women to appreciate about this venerable organization. Founded as a mail-order condom catalog, Adam & Eve has fought the good fight for First-Amendment rights all over the country and provides financial support for zero population growth worldwide. The company's Web site also hosts pages for Candida Royalle's Femme line of erotic videos "from a woman's perspective" (see p. 67) and the Sinclair Institute's *Better Sex* videos—you've probably seen ads in national magazines and newspapers for these educational videos about enhancing partner sex.

Prices are reasonable, particularly video prices; Adam & Eve co-produces many adult videos and currently finances and distributes both Candida Royalle's Femme line and Nina Hartley's educational sex videos. While the site's layout is cumbersome and slow-moving (only four products and photos per page), it includes a search function that allows surfers to call up a list of product recommendations by selecting the desired category and price range. Online ordering is secure, and you can order a free print catalog online (bear in mind that Adam & Eve will sell your name unless you specifically request they not do so). The return policy, more generous than most, offers a refund on any products (excluding videos) returned within ninety days.

For entertainment, check out this week's written installment of the site's "Dadahouse," an "erotic soap opera" (but you have to buy the CD-ROM to access the accompanying video clips). Or visit the "Ladies of a Risqué Business," featuring R-rated photos of and interviews with starlets such as Adam & Eve's current "spokesmodel," Juli Ashton. The interviews are long, interesting, and surprisingly revealing (Asia Carerra nakedly exposes her insecurities and near-pathological perfectionism). Access to more "spicy" pictures is available for a monthly fee.

Blowfish: Good Products for Great Sex

http://www.blowfish.com

The veteran site for online sales of sexual products, Blowfish got its start way back in 1994 (prehistory when it comes to the Web) as part of an Internet listserv—now it's a bustling emporium of over one thousand products.

Blowfish is clearly the lovechild of hip, queer San Franciscans, but shoppers of "all genders, persuasions, orientations, and varieties of relationships" will benefit from the proprietors' enthusiasm and literacy regarding sexual products. They offer up the "Fish Stories" column of informational tidbits, opinionated recommendations, and funny, chatty blurbs; as founder Christophe Pettus comments, "Our point of view is that of a kinky friend— or your really cool older sister or brother who's telling you what the 'in' sex products are."

The site features a comprehensive range of toys (including some specialty S/M and electric play items), books, magazines, comix, and videos. While not every product is accompanied by a photo, all have long, informative descriptions. You can reference the alphabetical indexes for books and videos, or use the site's search function to get to the page of products you're seeking. Online ordering is secure, and you can request a free print catalog online.

Come As You Are

http://www.comeasyouare.com

Modeled after the Good Vibrations toy store, this Canadian online shop is cooperatively-run and features an excellent selection of toys, books, and videos presented with humor and good taste. Come As You Are prides itself on being disability-positive; the site includes tips on adapting toys to accommodate certain disabilities, and an icon denotes particularly versatile toys. Visitors can learn more about the Canadian vendors who craft many of the toys, read Canadian trivia, and enjoy the humorous reviews, such as this description of a line of realistic dildos called Her Majesty's Men: "We may have distanced ourselves from the monarchy in practice, but in spirit we still love our queens, um queen. It doesn't matter what gender you fancy, these uber-realistic rubber dildos can be your man." Online ordering is not secure, but you can phone, fax, or mail in your order.

Dr. Susan Block's Journal

http://www.drsusanblock.com

If Jackie Collins or Judith Krantz were to stretch their imaginations to the limit, they still could never devise a character as utterly, irrepressibly off the wall as Dr. Susan Block, the beauty and brains behind the Dr. Susan Block Institute for the Erotic Arts and Sciences. Sex therapist, call-in radio hostess, cable-TV star, author, and all-around bon vivant, Dr. Block lives with her faithful aristocratic husband Maximillian and a rotating bevy of beauties known as "the Blockettes" at the Villa Piacere in the Hollywood Hills.

The sheer size of her six-hundred-page site makes it somewhat confusing to navigate, and her unusual range of product and professional endorsements are equally over-the-top (Dr. Block plugs everyone from Al Goldstein of *Screw* to her very own dentist and hairdresser to her telephone sex therapy services—available for a fee twenty-four hours a day!). However, it's well worth perusing the latest edition of her frequently updated "Private Journal of Pleasure, Art, Sex, Culture and Politics," which serves as a veritable who's-who and what's-what of "ethical hedonism." In her famed cable-TV shows (the audio version is accessible on her site), Dr. Block invites a panoply of female sex stars—from porn stars Nina Hartley and Sarah-Jane Hamilton to sex educators Carol Queen and Joani Blank—into her bed (literally) to chat and occasionally frolic seductively on camera. Volumes from her video series *The Encyclopedia of Sex and Fetish*, recommended books such as her own *Ten Commandments of Pleasure*, and an assortment of sex toys and lingerie are for sale on her site, but we were disappointed that neither online ordering nor a toll-free number are offered. The site also includes a chat room and a subscription-only area for an intimate look at the ladies of the Villa Piacere.

Oh, and don't forget to read Dr. Block's impassioned plea for the preservation of Zaire's endangered bonobo chimpanzees, beloved to her "because they use sex to create and maintain peace in their societies."

Renaissance Discovery International

http://www.sexhealth.org/shop/welcome.htm

A division of the Spencer Institute's Sexual Health Infocenter (see p.100), located in Montreal, Canada, Renaissance Discovery has a stated policy not to "sell products which may be considered harmful, illegal, exploitative, or overtly pornographic. Product selections are based entirely on their value in the promotion of sexual health, sexual education, self-help, and sensuality." Not surprisingly, this policy, which is probably the result of strict Canadian customs laws, limits the number of products in each category, but this online catalog offers a quality assortment of vibrators, dildos, anal toys, books, and videos—including a line of silicone toys imported from Germany. The "code of ethics" forswearing the sale of anything pornographic means that you'll find very little written erotica and no erotic videos. And, perhaps because of the difficulties of currency adaption, this international site doesn't sell electric vibrators.

Product presentation is simple and easy to navigate; in a nice feature, each product description includes a mention of its status (in stock or not) and return guarantee. Other pluses include the general information and selection tips provided for each category and reasonable prices. Online ordering is secure.

SensualSource

http://www.sensualsource.com

SensualSource, "a private site for the sexually curious," is an online boutique that presents quality products with all the confident style of a Body Shop or Patagonia. Boomer consumers are encouraged to let "us help you purchase the right experience for you." Its self-satisfied gloss aside, SensualSource does deliver the goods: accurate, well-researched information, a good selection of quality toys, books, and videos—which can be accessed from any area of the site—and secure online ordering. This is also the host site for *Libido* magazine and the Fantasy Photo Gallery (see p. 43).

The "Safer Sex Play Info" and "Sexual Health Advice" sections each contain a database of advice organized in a Q&A format; the former addresses the relative riskiness of different sexual activities, and the latter answers common questions regarding sex therapy, sexual response, and sexual problems. If your question remains unanswered after scrolling through the voluminous database, you can, for a fee, request individualized advice via e-mail to a husband-and-wife team of clinical sexologists. As one more bonus, we recommend the site's brief, well-written essays about how to identify secure servers and the use of "cookies," as well as a summary of available options for restricting children's access to adult materials.

Our only real beef with this site is its layout, which suffers from an excessive use of frames. The screen is broken up into so many pieces that the information you most want to see (answers to questions, descriptions of products) is crammed into a teeny, tiny frame—hey, we can't be the only boomers whose eyesight is failing!

Xandria Collection

http://www.xandria.com

The Xandria Collection has been in the mail-order business for over twenty years, and you've probably seen the company's ads, under the name "Lawrence Research Group," in many mainstream magazines. Check the "Sex Education" section for a nice concise history of sex toys and a good discussion of sexual response. You can also read the results of the 1997 National Sexual Health Survey documenting American sex toy habits, which was sponsored in part by Xandria. More information, entertainment, and a chat room are available to members.

The online Xandria Catalog takes the unusual tack of grouping products by either "category" or "benefit." Benefits include "Couples Searching for Excitement" or "Of Interest to Solo Women." Needless to say, there's plenty of product overlap among all these sections, but the sections "Of Interest to Gay Men" and "Of Interest to Gay Women" give the online catalog a more explicitly inclusive feel than the print catalog has. There's also an index listing every one of the several hundred items in the catalog in alphabetical order, and—presumably for those holding a catalog in their hands—there's a search function by product name or number. You can order Xandria's several different print catalogs online for a fee.

You'll find a wide range of battery vibrators, dildos, books, audios, lingerie, and soft-core and educational videos. Unfortunately, the "Better Sex Through Science" category promotes a number of herbal potency supplements of dubious scientific value. Online ordering is secure, or you can order by calling their toll-free number; both English- and Spanish-speaking operators are standing by. Xandria's prices are higher than their competitors'. However, in a business that is notoriously skittish about returns, Xandria stands out for its generous policy of replacing defective products for up to one year and taking back any product except videos and audiotapes—no questions asked—within sixty days.

BOOKS AND VIDEOS

Eros Comix

http://www.eroscomix.com

Slick and irreverent, this online catalog for one of the leading adult comix companies pulls no punches with breathless promises to deliver "all-out filth you'll have to see to believe." But somehow it's difficult to get offended by tongue-in-cheek copy encouraging you to "enter graphic filth" (accompanied by a sound clip of a woman's scream), or reassuring you that "if it's perverted, it's here" (accompanied by a sound clip of a sheep bleating).

Most of Eros's line appears on these pages, and you can enjoy a full-screen sample page from each comic. This is a great way to get a sense of the wide range of styles available in the ever-growing field of adult comix. Categories include "Manga" (Japanese erotic comix, redrawn here to include material censored in Japan), "Bondage," "Smut," and "Graphic Novels" from around the world. Online ordering is secure, and you can request a free print catalog online. Visitors can enjoy interactive puzzles and games, along with a chat room in which to shoot the breeze with other comix aficionados.

EroSpirit Research Institute

http://www.erospirit.org

" If you are on an erotic-spiritual path, this may be the Web page of your dreams," says Joseph Kramer, the driving force behind this "think tank for queer ecstatics." Kramer, a former Jesuit, is now a bodyworker, educator, and videographer. His attractive site offers you the opportunity to read articles about erotic spirituality, explore links to related sites, and shop for audiotapes and videos covering erotic massage, sacred prostitution,

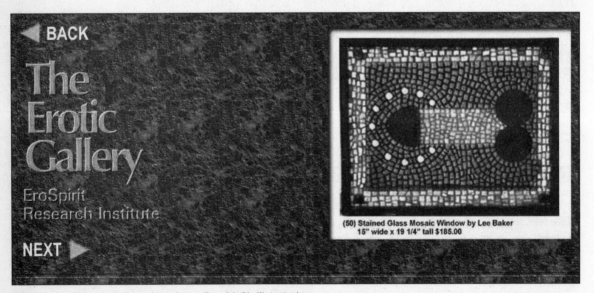

(50) Stained Glass Mosaic Window by Lee Baker
15" wide x 19 1/4" tall $185.00

Mosaic by Lee Baker http://www.the-park.com/Erospirit/Phallic/art14.htm

shamanic sex magic, and genital massage—plus more information on anal massage than you can shake a stick at (a well-lubricated stick with a flared base, of course). Photo stills for many of the videos are included. Online ordering is not secure. While the focus of this site is on queer sexuality, these videos are of interest to men and women of all persuasions. Kramer's "Fire on the Mountain: A Guide to Male Genital Massage," which depicts sex between two men, has been a best-seller with Good Vibrations's female customers since it's been on the market.

Much of the artwork from EroSpirit's now defunct "Phallic Art Gallery" remains posted on its server site, The Park (see the URL listed below the graphic on p. 144). This gorgeous museum-quality collection of phallic art pieces from all ages and cultures is a visual love song to the penis that will make you want to stand up and salute!

Excalibur Films

http://excaliburfilms.com

Granted, you'll need a good sense of humor to surf this site, home to thirty thousand adult videos (literally thousands are added to the inventory daily), along with DVDs and CD-ROMs. After all, the vast majority of the thousands of videos on display are pure trash. Maybe you, like us, will doubt that the power behind this thirty-five-year-old mail-order company is *really* a buxom blonde named Virginia Beaver (but then, people often think our last names aren't real either!). But this site is a treasure trove of every available adult video offered at unbeatable prices and backed up by a full return policy. Clearly, the Web is the perfect venue to handle a database of Excalibur's size. The site's excellent search function allows you to look up videos by director, company, star, and title. If you're overwhelmed by the selection, you can order a free print catalog online.

If you're a fan of adult video, this is the place to come for the best bargains on every release. Certain portions of the site (photos, movie reviews, and chat) are technically "members-only," but membership is free to anyone who has purchased an Excalibur video within the past year.

Focus International

http://www.focusint.com

Focus International is a distributor and producer of sex education, self-help, and therapy videos that has been in business since the early '70s. This online catalog gathers together some of the best informational sex videos in existence, from widely advertised titles such as the *Better Sex* series to harder-to-find titles on topics such as vaginismus, becoming orgasmic, and sex and aging. The site is no-frills in design, but despite the absence of an index or adequate information about the company, it remains a unique resource. Online ordering is secure, and you can request a free print catalog online.

Greenery Press

http://www.bigrock.com/~greenery

"Publishing responsible nonfiction about alternative sexualities," Greenery Press specializes in funny, heartfelt, inclusive sex books that will never make it to the airport bookstore. Titles like *A Hand in the Bush* (a guide to vaginal fisting) and *The Ethical Slut* are among the publisher's best-sellers, along with excellent guides to BDSM and more. Author bios, related articles, excellent resources, and Lady Green's own newsletter "for women and men exploring female dominance" round out the site, which is presented with impeccable simplicity, clarity, and good taste. Online ordering is not secure, and a toll-free number is available for those who'd prefer to order offline.

Passion Press

http://www.passionpress.com

This attractive, simple site displays the entire roster of a small production company specializing in audio erotica. The Passion Press line of about two dozen titles is divided between classics of Victorian smut, modern fiction such as the *Herotica* series, and nonfiction. The company also distributes "cyborgasm virtual audios," featuring 3-D recording technology. Reviews, customer comments, and interviews with performers enhance the product descriptions. Online ordering is not secure, but a toll-free number is provided, and you can request a free catalog online.

QSM

http://www.qualitysm.com

QSM stands for Quality S/M, and this mail-order company is "dedicated to bringing quality written material and education to the S/M community throughout the world." Their entire catalog of over five hundred books, magazines, and comics is posted on the site, and while their free print catalog comes out only a few times a year, the online version is updated monthly.

Best of all, excerpts are included from nearly every book for your browsing pleasure. Alas, online ordering is not available, but a toll-free number is.

Don't leave the site without checking out QSM's quarterly class schedule. Even if you can't make the classes, which are held in San Francisco, we guarantee that the descriptions of seminars on "terror and kidnap scenes" or "the art of sensuous spanking" will spark your imagination. An excellent "Kink Links" section points the way to reliable publications, shopping resources, professional dominants, and BDSM organizations. Finally, the "Ask Mistress Flora" advice column offers a taste of the site's good-humored attitude: "QSM reserves the right to edit questions for clarity, brevity, or just to prove who's the Top. All questions become the property of QSM, and if a Hollywood studio offers a movie deal, we intend to retire in style."

BDSM AND FETISH

Adam and Gillian's Sensual Whips and Toys

http://www.catalog.com/utopian/www/whips.html

There's more to the wide world of whips than many of us could have imagined, and this well-organized online catalog gives you the skinny on every conceivable strap, flogger, paddle, cane, and cat. Adam and Gillian have been designing whips and toys since 1987, and their enthusiasm for S/M and dedication to craftsmanship shine through in comments such as this: "These items are designed, crafted and "feel-tested" here in our workshop. . . . We stand in front of everything we make—at least once—and then stand behind it the rest of the year."

Presentation is simple and the site is easy to navigate; each category of products is laid out on one page with short, but informative, text about individual items; group photos of the products are quick to load and allow you to compare their size and shape easily. You're encouraged to design the implement of your dreams at no extra charge by custom-blending the features you desire. Unfortunately, the site doesn't offer online ordering, but those who do place an order via phone, fax, and mail can count on reasonable prices and a one-year warranty. You can also order a print catalog online for a fee.

Adam and Gillian's umbrella site, the Utopian Network, hosts the Web page for *The Sandmutopian Guardian*, a.k.a. "the *Popular Mechanics*™ of kinky sex." Here you'll find information on subscribing to this quarterly print magazine for the S/M community, writers' guidelines, and a comprehensive index to all the subject matter in previous issues—but sadly, none of the articles or reviews from the magazine itself.

Axfords Corset Catalogue

http://www.axfords.com

Since 1880, Axfords has been designing and manufacturing this "essential item in any self-respecting sexual sophisticate's wardrobe," and this very British company has thousands of corsets in stock to fit women and men alike. The site offers a wonderful history of corsets, a brief discussion of corsets and sex ("restricting your waist needn't restrict your imagination"), and a complete catalog of corsets, bloomers, and other undergarments modeled by a bevy of natural-looking British lasses—after one image too many of fetish-clad babes in dungeons, these photos of corseted damsels playing croquet in the sunshine are a novel treat indeed. Online ordering is secure, and you can order Axfords's sixty-four-page print catalog online for a fee. A handy currency converter on the site will help you calculate what you owe.

Chainmail & More: Fantasies in Metal

http://www.sblades.com

Many of our survey respondents recommended this charming site, which features a line of custom-made chainmail fashions, jewelry, manacles, collars, and piercing decorations crafted by a couple named Sunshyn and Greger. These two are clearly proud of their handiwork and provide detailed explanations of their materials and techniques, including Sunshyn's animation page, which presents tips for working with chainmail. All products are displayed in thumbnail photos, which can be viewed full-screen. We particularly like the regular guys and gals modeling the products (regular in a biker kind of way). Online ordering is secure, and you can request a print catalog online for a fee. Check out the links to gothic and fantasy sites, including a site purveying customized vampire fangs.

DivaWeb

http://www.divaweb.com

This San Francisco-based boutique showcases fetish fashions, bondage gear, and related art pieces, videos, books, magazines, and CD-ROMs that hail from all over the United States and Europe. What's particularly pleasing about the site is that it provides access to information and images from dozens of cottage designers and small manufacturers, whose merchandise you wouldn't be likely to find without traveling to some pretty remote byways. Even if you're not in the market for a corset, six-inch stilettos, a bondage belt, or a spanking magazine, you're bound to appreciate the gorgeous photographic imagery on this site. And if you are ready to buy, all products are for sale either through Diva Web's secure server or from their print catalog, which you can order for a fee online. This site is also the home of *Diva Z*, an e-zine devoted to the fetish club scene. The site is accessible through Netscape, but it looks best with Microsoft Explorer.

The Frugal Domme

http://www.frugaldomme.com

"Why buy it when you can make it?" is webmistress Domina's motto, followed by "If you can't make it, for heaven's sake, buy it as cheap as possible!" And true to her word, the Frugal Domme offers canes, floggers, sensual toys such as fur mitts, medical items, and more—all at excellent prices and all clearly and simply presented. The site also features a wide and witty range of information compiled from a variety of sources: etiquette tips for D/S play online and off; the "Ask Domina" advice column; FAQs on precautions to take during D/S play; and links to BDSM resources. A unique aspect of the site is its lovingly assembled set of links to an impressive array of do-it-yourself tips, including instructions on assembling a birch bundle and improvising sex toys with items found in your kitchen or hotel room. As yet, you can only order via snail mail or e-mail, but after reading through the wealth of content on the site, we think you should be grateful to make the extra effort (and we're sure Domina agrees). A print catalog, which has fewer products than the online catalog, is available for a fee.

Morgan's Toybox

http://www.charm.net/~morgans

Ann and Morgan—a self-described "D&S couple" who met on a BBS (a computer bulletin board), moved across the country to settle together in Maryland, and now moonlight as fetish manufacturers—are the charming entrepreneurs behind this cottage industry of leather crafts and toys. Morgan was inspired to start his own line of inexpensive S/M toys after purchasing one too many shoddy items (a whip handle came apart in the car before he even got home from the store). With endearing candor, he writes, "I hope I can entice you with prices that will enhance your toy bag and my next mortgage payment."

And indeed, the prices for his line of restraints, collars, whips, paddles, crops, clamps, cock-and-ball toys, and more are extremely reasonable (shipping is free for most orders). Product illustrations are simple black-and-white line drawings; blurbs are lengthy and informational; and helpful hints abound regarding both product selection and safety tips. Online ordering is not secure, but a toll-free number is provided as an option.

Skin Two

http://www.skintwo.co.uk/clothing

Whether you've got a yen to order custom-made latex and PVC clothing or just want to look at the pictures, you'll enjoy browsing the online clothing catalog from London's famed fetish clothing manufacturer. This beautifully designed site makes intelligent use of frames. You select the product area you're interested in—men's or women's latex and men's or women's PVC—and thumbnails come up in one screen. When you click on the thumbnail of your choice, the photo comes up at two-thirds screen, along with product specifications and ordering information. The photos aren't explicit, but they're definitely arousing in a sleek, sassy *Vogue* magazine way—and what a treat to see gorgeous women *and* men slicked up in rubber.

Online ordering is not secure. Print catalogs are available for a fee (understandable since the opulence of the work by photographers such as Trevor Watson renders them more like coffee-table books than catalogs). Catalogs are just one part of Skin Two's "comprehensive interactive fetish Web site," where members have access to an e-zine, galleries of photos and art, and message boards.

Stockroom/JT Toys

http://www.stockroom.com/catalog.htm

This pioneering adult company has been purveying sex and bondage toys online since the late '80s. The Stockroom manufactures its own products in Los Angeles, and its extensive assortment of reasonably priced S/M toys is the primary reason to visit the site. A standard array of battery vibrators, rubber dildos, books, and videos rounds out their selection. Online ordering is secure.

The presentation is bare-bones; products are described in laundry-list format and illustrated with black-and-white photos. But this site has a nice community feel, and it is updated daily with specials and sale items. There's a chat room and a photo gallery of images from previous print catalogs (the print catalog is available free with orders, or for a fee). The Stockroom also sponsors a site we particularly enjoyed: Akasha's Web presents the philosophical musings and S/M erotica of an unabashed femdom (you'll find it on their excellent links page).

S P E C I A L T Y

Condom Sense

http://www.condoms.net

An example of online marketing at its best, Condom Sense not only offers name-brand condoms, lubricants, and other safer-sex products at rock-bottom prices but also offers excellent advice and information to support the philosophy that we should all "enjoy sex and use condom sense!" While the product selection is not as extensive as that of emporiums such as Condomania, the folks at Condom Sense provide a good sampling of the best safer-sex supplies currently available, as well as ample information to

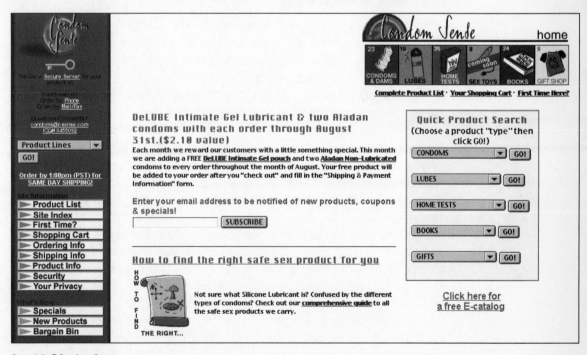

Copyright©Condom Sense

guide you in making your selection, including a search function and charts that make it easy to view the features of each brand of condoms at a glance. The entire site is attractive, well designed, and easy to navigate. Best of all, you simply can't beat these prices; as former wholesalers, the folks at Condom Sense skip the middleman to bring you great deals (including free shipping). Online ordering is secure, and customer satisfaction is guaranteed with a money-back return policy.

Condom Sense encourages customer interaction with a predominantly twenty-something clientele, sponsoring monthly drawings for free gifts, the cheeky but sensitive "Don't Ask Michelle" (or DAM) advice column, and customer polls asking questions such as "Would you use a male pill?" or "Do you use protection during oral sex?" A chat room is in the works. We especially admire the site's archive of general sex- and health-related news items, which includes a search function and postings of the Centers for Disease Control's daily AIDS summary.

Condomania

http://www.condomania.com

Condomania was the first company to take condoms out from behind drugstore counters and put them into a boutique environment, and it has been in the retail and mail-order business since 1991. The Starbucks of condom stores, their playful motto is "When you get busy, we get busy."

As you'd expect, what you'll find on this five-hundred-page site are condoms, condoms, condoms—over three hundred brands, along with lubricants and novelties. The site also features general safer-sex information in the form of well-researched, if slightly pedestrian, lectures and links to a variety of health and safer-sex organizations. Presentation is strongest in the product sections, where thorough information and silhouettes of condoms side by side allow you to compare and contrast possible purchases. The nifty "Condom Wizard" takes you through a series of questions designed to help you narrow down which condom will best suit your needs and tastes. Fortunately, a search function is also available for those who already know what they're looking for—since there is no index of all the products for sale. In fact, the entire site suffers a bit from the "Are we there yet?" syndrome, and you have to click through numerous pages to reach your destination. Online ordering is secure, and you can request a free catalog online. Prices are not as good as those of Condom Sense, but the selection is wider.

Real Doll

http://www.realdoll.com

Perhaps you find yourself wondering from time to time, Gosh, if they can put a man on the moon, why can't they make a truly realistic love doll? Perhaps not. Either way, anyone who appreciates the truly surreal or has a soft spot for American ingenuity in all its manifestations will get a kick out of the Real Doll Web site. The Real Doll is a five-thousand-dollar solid-silicone "lovetoy," manufactured (you guessed it) in Southern California and marketed exclusively online. All the features and options of several different styles of Real Dolls are presented in earnest detail. For five thousand dollars, you do get to select hair color, body shape, and even pubic hair styling, along with three possible "entries" (vaginal, anal, or oral). Don't forget to check out the video animation demonstrating the elasticity of Real Doll's silicone breasts, and don't despair: a male real doll is in development. A select list of links to other robot- and mannequin-related sex sites rounds out the site.

Tantra.com

http://www.tantra.com

This attractive woman-owned site offers resources, information, and products related to tantra and sacred sexuality. You'll find introductory essays defining tantra, a complete national directory of tantra teachers and workshops, articles and excerpts from many of the books sold through the site, free personal ads, links to a variety of sexuality and relationship sites, and more. The Q&A section, answered by a rotating roster of tantra experts, ostensibly focuses on sacred sexuality, but the questions are charmingly generic—for example, "Why won't my boyfriend give me oral sex?" or "How can I delay ejaculation?" Apparently, even the enlightened must come to grips with these age-old questions!

The site's E-Sensuals catalog contains a couple of toys, lubes, audios, and CDs, but it is most notable for its comprehensive selection of books and videos related to sex and spirituality. Online ordering is secure, and you can request a free print catalog online. There's also a search function for the entire site.

Chapter Seven

Online Rendezvous

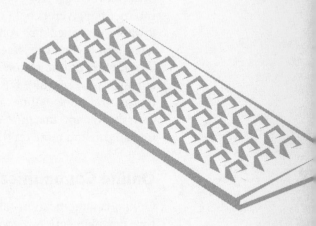

By now you've gotten the message loud and clear: the Web is an amazing resource for information, entertainment, and services. So we could speculate that fifty million Americans are headed online simply because they're thrilled to be able to review their bank balances, e-mail their far-flung families, order airline tickets, and check the weather reports on the other side of the country. We could suggest that at this very minute droves of women and men are surfing the Internet, muttering to themselves: "Gosh, this puts that old *Encyclopedia Brittanica* of mine to shame!" But that wouldn't be the whole story. People are spending their time online *talking* to one another—and they're talking about sex.

In this chapter, we'll give you a brief tour of the ways in which you can reach out and just about touch someone on the Web. And we'll share some true-life tales of love, lust, intimacy, and friendships forged online—relationships that often cross over into "RL," or real life. As one of our many survey respondents who raved about the life-transforming effects of online communication testifies, "Being online has allowed me to explore my sexuality in a safely anonymous environment; my online friends—who have since become my RL friends too—have helped me work through many issues in my life and have brought me a lot of joy!"

Over the past few years, online sex chat—especially the mutually arousing encounters that are commonly referred to as "cybersex"—has been the focus of much media hand-wringing over its "addictive" powers, the marriages that have been destroyed as a result of cyberaffairs, and the possibility of being duped or harmed by online Don Juans and Doña Juanas who aren't what they pretend to be. Yet, for every harrowing tale of deceit and betrayal, there's a story of newfound confidence, friendship, and love. The Internet has given people the ability to flirt, role-play, and communicate in a whole new medium—one that is characterized by a liberating sense of safety, self-acceptance, freedom from inhibition, and above all, playfulness. We think of online communication as a tool—like any good sex toy, it can enhance your sex life, but the basic ingredients of a satisfying encounter remain the same online and off. Memorable sex of any variety requires curiosity, humor, imagination, self-knowledge, and empathy. You just might find all this and more on the Web.

Online Communication: Let Me Count the Ways

Online communication takes two basic forms: real time or delayed. Real-time communication is commonly referred to as "chat," since the exchange of typed comments is instantaneous and impermanent, as in real-life conversations. Chat isn't necessarily saved or recorded, although it is possible to log transcripts, if you wish. Alternately, you can participate in the "slow-motion" conversations of conferences, in which everyone who participates in a particular discussion reads and posts messages sequentially. Participants

---

CHAT CHARM

Mind your manners online, and you're guaranteed to make friends and influence people.

• When you first enter a chat room or conference, "lurk" a while (i.e., read the discussion before diving in with your own contributions) to get a sense of the group's general tone.

• If you don't understand what's going on or how to handle certain technical details, read the site's FAQ section. It was written and posted in order to preempt unnecessary questions.

• Keep it short, sweetie! Time is money online, and you should strive to keep your comments concise and on subject (of course, if you're engaged in an erotic dialog, it may be perfectly appropriate to ramble a bit).

• Don't correct other people's typos. Everyone is typing too fast to bother with niceties like capitalizing words or correcting spelling. On the other hand, you'd better keep a grip on your grammar if you want to get your point across.

• Don't "spam" or fire off so many messages in a row that you disrupt the discussion.

• Don't use all caps—it's as rude as shouting.

• Don't believe everything you read.

can show up hours or days after a message on a certain topic is posted and add their own two cents.

In short, chat is like mingling at a party, and conferencing is like corresponding with many people at once. Both chat and conferencing can be used to contact like-minded individuals from around the world. Online communication has proven to be a particular boon to members of marginalized communities—gay teens, transgendered individuals, folks in polyamorous relationships, and S/M practitioners—who find the support, information, and solidarity online that can be in short supply offline. You yourself may find you prefer one or the other mode of communication, or you may enjoy each at different times for different reasons.

Conferencing

Usenet

Online conferencing has been around for close to twenty years. Before the Web existed, there was Usenet: a network of Unix computers that linked techies from around the world and enabled them to post messages to one another on a variety of different Internet discussion boards or newsgroups. Needless to say, the ins and outs of Unix did not remain the sole compelling topic for long, and as more and more people gained access to the Internet and mastered Unix commands, newsgroups related to sex multiplied like bunnies. Usenet groups are sorted into several general categories, characterized by prefixes such as "alt," indicating alternative or unusual topics, "rec," indicating recreation, and "soc," indicating social issues. The "alt" category quickly became a vast repository of sex-related materials, featuring conference topics ranging from "alt.sex.anal" to "alt.sex.zoophilia," an outpouring of erotic writing, and numerous binary files containing photos and graphics. (In fact, many of the nudie pix that are featured on adult pay sites are simply swiped from Usenet.)

Ah, but nothing stays the same, and in recent years the alt.sex newsgroups have fallen prey to the scourge of spamming, which means that in order to find the good stuff, you, gentle reader, would have to wade through an ocean of X-rated ads, get-rich-quick scams, and anguished flames declaring that you will BURN IN HELL for your prurient interests. Resourceful regulars from spammed-out groups have created new moderated groups, in which spam is filtered out. Best of all, Usenet newsgroups are no longer accessible only to the Internet cognoscenti. Most browsers come with a "newsreader" function that allows you to read and post to newsgroups, and there are a number of Web sites devoted to archiving the best of newsgroups for posterity.

Boards, Boards, Boards

Whether they go under the name of bulletin boards, discussion boards, message boards, or forums, these non-Usenet conferences are designed to allow for more leisurely—and ostensibly more thoughtful—discussions than you'll find in chat rooms. When you visit a conference, you'll find a list of different topics, from the exquisitely particular ("Best Songs/Music About Sex") to the sweepingly vague ("Issues and Debates in Human Sexuality"). Once you select the topic that interests you, you'll be able to view a series of messages, the number of responses each posted message has generated, and the date and time of the most recent posting. To read messages, simply point and click on the posting that intrigues you, and then continue reading as many in the thread of responses as you like. It's equally easy to attach your own comments.

Conferences are cropping up all over the Web, and you've probably noticed that many of the sites reviewed in this book feature their own message boards. This medium can't be beat as a simple, nonintimidating way of getting your feet wet in online communication. Whether you're contributing your own oral sex tips on Isadora Alman's Sexuality Forum, flirting on A Dyke's World Pillowtalk forum, or commiserating over someone's relationship travails on the Thrive Passion boards, you'll learn firsthand just how easy it is to make a personal connection in cyberspace. What's truly revolutionary about these conferences is that people are sharing authentic details of their sex lives. We're not saying that the minute you get online you'll suddenly shed all your anxieties about sexual discourse or your concerns about being perceived as "normal" in your tastes and talents. But the combination of the total anonymity of the Web and the wide range of sexual possibilities it provides is profoundly uninhibiting.

Although conferences aren't, strictly speaking, taking place in real time, many—such as Isadora's Sexuality Forum, Bianca's Smut Shack, and the WELL—boast such dedicated and active participants that you can essentially "hang out" online swapping messages with your pals. However, conferences lack some aspects of chat's immediate gratification: you can't send a private message to another conference user through the system, as you can in a chat room, and by and large, members of a conference are there to talk about sex, not to have it. In fact, in a thriving community it's not at all unusual for a conference thread that started on a sexual topic to veer off into topics as diverse as grammar, car repair, or resumé tips—just because people are talking about things that usually go unsaid in daily life doesn't mean that they stop talking about everything else.

E-mail

Now, what if you meet a stranger across a crowded conference room whose postings seem to be the smartest, most compelling commentary you've ever read? Or what if he or she just sounds kinda cute? There's no reason you can't make the transition to a one-on-one conversation via personal e-mail. Thanks to the explosion in online communication, several sites (notably Hotmail and Yahoo!) offer free, anonymous e-mail, so you can exchange communiqués with complete confidentiality.

The Dating Game

If you're seeking a real-life companion, not just an erotic pen pal, you might want to head over to a dating site. Dating sites apply a high-tech veneer to some old-fashioned matchmaking techniques. You submit a personal profile in which you specify what you're looking for in a partner. Then your cyberyenta searches every name in the site's enormous database to find those that are your match in terms of geography, personality, and attitude. You can communicate with as many of these lovely bachelors and bachelorettes as you desire in complete safety—most dating sites offer anonymous e-mail services. The "full service" sites also offer chat rooms, advice columns, and testimonials from happy, hitched couples. Some sites charge a monthly fee, while others are free.

Matchmaking sites tend to cater to individuals seeking long-term relationships, so if you're looking for someone to have fun with, rather than walk down the aisle with, you might want to seek out online personal ads. As this survey respondent comments, they provide a nearly effortless way to cast a wide net:

> The uncensored personal ads on Yahoo are even more interesting than those in newspapers. Online dating is much quicker and less painful than regular dating; I feel more in control, and it's very safe. I can respond to six personal ads easily in an evening, and if all these men write back, we can begin conversations that same night—within two or three messages I can generally determine if I want the conversations to continue. I couldn't very easily pack six dates into one week, even if I had the opportunity to try.

Of course, as another respondent indicates, a greater pool of applicants sometimes just means you have to exhibit extra perseverance:

> I met the man of my life from an ad on a big, beautiful women's personals site. We fell for each other via e-mail, met two weeks after he responded to my post, and have been inseparable ever since. This said, I chose him out of some three hundred men who responded. Most were clearly not as they portrayed themselves to be. Many were married. Others were simply not people I'd ever be interested in communicating with, let alone dating. Out of three hundred some-odd guys, I replied to less than a dozen via e-mail, met six in person, and easily chose my guy the moment he showed up in my virtual mailbox.

WHAT WOMEN WANT

"I love reading about sexual things. When I know that the writer is thinking of me specifically, it is completely, absolutely thrilling. And when I find someone who enjoys the same level of explicitness I do and has similar writing skills, it's particularly alluring."

Real-Time Chat

While folks have been conferencing back and forth about sex for decades now, it took the development of real-time chat to bring the phenomenon into the mainstream and before the media's rapt gaze. Who doesn't know by now that the subscription base of commercial online services such as AOL, CompuServe, and Prodigy is founded on chat? Most notably, AOL's membership rocketed into the millions by the late '90s, thanks to dirty talkers all across the nation. The easy interface of AOL chat rooms, and their guaranteed anonymity—members can create up to five different "profiles" or identities for themselves—have emboldened countless men and women to stay up until the wee hours exchanging flirtatious and provocative comments.

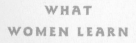

Given the huge success of AOL's chat rooms (over fifteen thousand strong), it's no surprise that canny Web site developers have turned their attention to creating Web-based chat systems. Now that the technology for chatting on the Web has gotten nearly as transparent and user-friendly as AOL's, sites such as Yahoo, Women's Wire, and Talk City nurture bustling chat rooms of their own. Of course, plenty of people are chatting about topics *other* than sex, but sex is basically the engine powering the chat locomotive. Chat rooms on both AOL and the Web frequently host scheduled events in which specific authors, experts, or speakers are available to chat with curious fans. You can query Susie Bright about her latest book, Gloria Brame about BDSM, or romance novelists about where their ideas come from. And best of all, most of these sites are free, so you can chat until dawn without paying a subscriber fee.

If you've never tried chat, or if you've only paid a brief, cursory visit to a chat room, you may well wonder how the heck anybody is getting off on this juvenile, badly spelled, poorly expressed drivel. It's true that, at first glance, chat room conversations can seem banal and relentlessly one-noteish. AOL is particularly infamous for the fact that any user with a feminine handle can be subjected to a tedious barrage of IMs (Instant Messages) containing cheesy queries along the lines of "R U horny?," "Let's party 2 night," or "Can you send me your picture?" As one survey respondent sums it up, "I've never found a chat room that rose above a sixth-grade level."

Certainly, the relatively brief and superficial comments you'll often find on public chat are far from compelling. However, as chat fans are quick to point out, aren't the majority of conversations you strike up offline pretty banal? Wherever you roam, you'll need to invest some time and energy in hooking up with interesting, like-minded people—casual one-line greetings can eventually lead to extended satisfying encounters, whether these are with fellow *Star Trek* fans, fellow gardeners, or fellow horny people! We'll review the ways in which you can make your chat experience a positive one in one of the sections that follows, but first we'll touch briefly on some other types of real-time communication.

Internet Relay Chat

More commonly known as IRC, Internet Relay Chat was developed in the late '80s in Finland to allow those with Internet access to connect on sort of a worldwide party line. It's a text-based form of chat (no exchanging photos here, folks) featuring thousands of different channels. And, just as you can find sexual materials galore on Usenet, on IRC channels you'll find erotic chat, S/M dungeons, and more. To participate in IRC, you need to download specific client software and then connect with an Internet server that is part of an IRC network.

In essence, the downside of IRC is that it requires a greater level of technical expertise than do other chat environments. The upsides are that IRC will introduce you to a vast virtual realm of channels on an extraordinary range of topics, anyone who wants to can start her or his own channel, and it's cheap! We've reviewed a couple of Web sites that provide more detailed advice and instruction on getting connected to one of the IRC networks, such as EFnet, DALnet, and UNDERnet.

ICQ

One fairly new piece of Internet software is ICQ (as in "I Seek You"), which puts Web-based instant messaging into the hands of anyone with Internet access. First, you create a list of your friends and colleagues who also have ICQ; then, whenever you connect to the Web, a panel pops up on your screen telling you which of them is online. You can send real-time messages back and forth or chat simultaneously with several users. And you can save a log of the chat. Obviously, this software has infinite possibilities, not just for business meetings or sports discussions, but for tender and torrid exchanges. Currently, it's still free.

MUDs

MUDs ("Multi-User Dimensions" or "Multi-User Dungeons") are text-based, interactive adventure games, in which multiple players role-play specified characters and navigate fantasy realms. The adventures can include battles, run-ins with Wizards, and—since real-time chat is involved—a fair bit of socializing and sex. To enter a MUD, you need to download specific client software and connect with the specific host server. We've listed a couple of sites that are good gateways to further information on exploring the wide world of MUDs, and their numerous variants—MOOs, MUSHes, and MUCKs.

What to Expect When You're Chatting

Probably the most important thing to keep in mind when you start out in chat is that you're in the driver's seat. You get to decide when you chat, with whom you chat, and what you chat about. Many of our survey respondents commented that online communication has helped them become more outgoing and confident offline. "I've gotten a little less inhibited," says one such respondent. "I've learned to censor myself less offline since my strong and open opinions have been so well-received online." It's arguable that there are precious few occasions when a woman feels in complete control of a sexual encounter, so it should come as no surprise that the opportunity to explore personal fantasies in utter safety has the potential to be a heady and powerfully transformative experience.

Getting Started

First things first: Put some thought into choosing your online name, or "handle." At this point, women are still a minority online, so they tend to attract a lot of attention in chat rooms and on IRC channels. If you want to

SAFE CYBERSEX

Remember the scene in *The Wizard of Oz* in which Dorothy and her pals tiptoe nervously through the forest chanting "Lions and tigers and bears—oh, my!"? Today's Internet novice might feel similarly apprehensive approaching the online world, thanks to the relentless stream of media reports about "stalkers and pedophiles and thieves." In reality, you're no more likely to encounter any of these antisocial characters online than in your everyday life, and while you may receive unwanted advances or harassing messages in an online environment, you have a wide array of coping mechanisms at your disposal. Here are a few simple things you can do to protect your privacy and ensure your safety online:

•Don't give out personal information to strangers, either online or over the phone. Use common sense when filling out a member profile in a chat room: don't include information that could be used to identify you offline. If someone claiming to be a representative of your ISP approaches you online requesting personal information, don't buy it! Similarly, if you get a phone call from someone claiming to be an employee of your ISP, ask for a name and number so you can return the call—and weed out scammers in the process. If the caller appears legitimate but is requesting personal information (such as your social security number) without adequate explanation, ask to speak to a supervisor, and persist until you get a satisfactory explanation.

•If someone is sending you unwanted messages, ignore them. Don't respond, or you risk revealing more information about yourself or giving your pesky correspondent reason to think that you're in some kind of reciprocal relationship. You nearly always have the option of filtering out unwanted messages. You can set your e-mail program to "kill" messages from e-mail addresses that you specify, thereby deleting them before cut down on the number of "R U Horny?" messages you'll be getting, select a gender-neutral or nonprovocative handle. The number of solicitations you receive will probably drop drastically once you change your handle from "Bunny" to "Susan." Of course, you may *want* to explore role-playing as "Blonde Bimbo," in which case, we salute you! In either case, most Web-based chat systems make it very easy for you to change your handle, so you can experiment with as many personae as you please.

Don't be deterred if you feel somewhat flustered the first time you enter a chat room. It can take a while to get the hang of the logistics. In fact, rather than diving right into a room called, say, "The Dungeon," you might want to practice your chops in a nonsex room. After a few chat sessions in a political action or reproductive rights room, you should be confident enough to exercise your rights to erotic free speech.

When you enter a chat room you'll be able to view the handles of all the other participants, although this list is ever-shifting as folks cruise in and out. The text of chat scrolls across your screen fairly quickly, and if you're in a crowded room it can be confusing to follow the thread of multiple conversations, but you'll soon learn to filter out those you're not interested in.

you even read them. In conferences, it's sometimes possible to filter out the postings of somebody you find obnoxious: his or her postings won't even appear on your screen. Most chat rooms and IRC channels feature an "ignore" command, so that you can block messages from whomever you select (alternately, on IRC you can make yourself "invisible" to anyone who's not on the same channel with you). However, if you're being consistently harassed or feel threatened, it's a good idea to accept (but not respond to) the messages and print them out as documentation that you can use in filing a complaint with your harasser's ISP or IRC operator.

•If you're ready to make the move from an online acquaintance to a real-life meeting, take some basic precautions. Communicate by phone a couple of times first just to make sure that "SweetSally" really is a she, or that "ClitLicker" is above the age of consent. Meet in a public place, make sure a friend knows where and when you're meeting your cyberpal, and if you're traveling out of town, make sure you have your own place to stay.

•For more information on protecting yourself online, check out the "Privacy Tips" sidebar on p. 198 as well as the following Web sites:

Katherine the Art Chick
Katherine offers these two pages:

http://www.io.com/~villyard/xcg
Provides tips on filtering unwanted mail.

http://www.io.com/~xcg/tips/irc.html
Visit this page to learn how to avoid harassment on IRC.

Grrltalk
http:/www.grrltalk.net
This lesbian chat site includes tips on avoiding harassment on IRC.

Online Harrassment Resources
http://www.io.com/~barton/harassment.html
General safety tips and harassment resources for women online.

Once you're engaged in a conversation with someone, you'll also learn to adjust to the slight overlap between your responses, as sometimes you'll both be typing simultaneously and may go off on different conversational tangents.

Do make a point of visiting the site's FAQ section so you can get an overview of the variety of commands available to you, such as how to send a private message, how to create a private room, and how to filter out the messages of somebody who's annoying you. These common commands are always designed to be extremely simple, usually involving a point and click.

Private or Public?

As the name would indicate, private rooms allow you to speak privately with whomever you invite into the room with you (on IRC, opening a DCC chat is the equivalent of creating a private room). Some people prefer private rooms for any kind of serious conversation or possible cybersex. Others enjoy the voyeuristic, exhibitionistic, or just plain sociable possibilities of public rooms. We'll let some of our survey respondents point out the pros and cons of each type of room:

> I enter public rooms when I'm interested in debating or general flirting. I prefer a private room for something more intimate and personal, because public rooms attract too many people who are only interested in disrupting other people's conversations with bad pick-up lines and borderline harassment.

> If you're really clicking in a public chat, and everyone stays quiet except for expressions of awe, that is a terrific feeling. The feeling of being on stage, but not being able to see the audience. Unforgettable.

> I prefer public chat rooms because I like to read what other people are doing. If you're in a private chat room and things are boring, it's really hard to move on to something else. Also, I like the idea of showing off for others.

R U Coming?

Of course, you can spend a lot of time in chat rooms simply talking about sex, but eventually you may want to *have* sex—to collaborate on a custom-crafted erotic scenario that inspires long-distance mutual masturbation. This is what people mean when they refer to "cybersex," or "cybering." If you've never tried it, cybersex can sound improbable, but you don't have to look too far to come up with analogous activities that you may already find quite appealing. As one survey respondent notes, "If you like erotic literature and phone sex, you'll like cybersex." It's all about flexing your brain to satisfy your libido.

We must admit that when we first started researching this chapter, our inquiring minds were haunted by one crucial question about cybersex: Is anybody *really* getting off? Are these folks actually having orgasms, or are they just typing their way to arousal and then taking care of business once they've logged off? As with every question related to human sexuality, the answer seems to be that some are, and some aren't. Here is a representative sampling of testimonials from sticky keyboards across the country:

I type with one hand and play with myself with the other. Sometimes I use a vibrator or other toy. When I say I am coming, I am. I believe the same has been true of my partners. I don't know why it works to engage this way, but it does.

It's too hard to beat off with a computer—I've tried. I can't scroll and masturbate at the same time very effectively. And I have a real tough time getting turned on while I'm typing.

It's just another way of masturbating—and not a good one for those who like "hands free" stimulation. However, I can attest that computer keyboards can withstand certain amounts of Astroglide lubricant!

I sometimes have better orgasms online than with live people. That's frustrating! Maybe it's because online sex is so focused.

Before we ever met in RL, my husband and I were flirting on a MUD. We were in a more-or-less private room and things got steamy. We told each other what we'd like to do and what we'd like to experience, and then carried it out. It was the only time I faked an orgasm with him.

You get pretty good at typing with one hand. There are a lot of times—especially when I'm having an orgasm, or the guy is, or both—that we just type "ooooooohooooooooooooooooooooo yeahoohoh hdfjsahloa dioiooooooooooooh yeah!!!!!!!" Just bashing hands randomly on the keyboard, which does not take a great deal of precision.

As that last respondent so vividly demonstrates, participants who craft elaborately worded scenarios to get each other's juices flowing have a lot more leeway when approaching the point of no return! Cybersex has its own language, with conventions that have evolved in order to add dimension to written communication. You may notice that chat can see-saw back and forth between the first and third person. Sometimes people communicate directly in the first person, and sometimes they essentially collaborate on an erotic narrative in the third person. Sometimes the use of handles (your handle appears in front of everything you type) leads to a unique blend of first and third person, for example, "SassySub lowers her eyes demurely as LadyJane bends me over her knee." It's common for people to compensate for the absence of body cues by drawing a picture with words, indicating gestures or physical movements in brackets, such as "[blush]" or "[grinning wickedly]." As a survey respondent comments, "It's almost as though you were reading erotica, except you are also writing the erotic story, and you don't know what's going to happen next."

R U Male or Female?

It's a widely reported fact that not everyone is what—or who—they appear to be online. After all, the anonymity of chat affords unparalleled opportunities for role-playing, so it hasn't taken long for boys to realize that they can be girls and girls to realize that they can be boys. However, at this stage of the game, far more men are passing as women than vice versa—and who can blame them? Women get all the attention in chat rooms, and if you're a men looking to craft an erotic scenario with another person, your odds of getting a response go up exponentially if you don't let on that you've got a penis. This has resulted in somewhat of a gender panic in chat rooms, as many men—horrified at the prospect of engaging in cyberhomosexuality—pepper anyone with a female handle with the question "R U female?"

As the following survey respondent indicates, when you engage in sex chat, you're collaborating on creating a fantasy. If part of your fantasy involves flirting and having sex as a member of the opposite sex, what's wrong with that? You are connecting through your imaginations, not through your bodies.

> I am interested in the brain I am talking to, and if that person chooses to be a certain gender, then dadgummit s/he *is* that gender when s/he is online. Part of my online policy is that I *never* ask what gender someone is . . . I *love* it when someone can keep me guessing.

While we salute anyone who wants to engage in a little online gender play, there are situations in which these deceptions are inappropriate and intrusive. For instance, some men are relentless about crashing women-only chat rooms to proposition, harass, or generally pester participants. As a result, if you visit a lesbian chat room, you can expect to be run through a battery of tests before being accepted as the gen-u-ine article and invited into the fold. You may be asked questions related to female clothing, menstrual cycles, and the like—including some questions that we ourselves would be hard-pressed to answer, such as "What size pantyhose do you

WHAT WOMEN LEARN

"I've learned how other people fantasize about sex. (It's not only me!)"

wear?" If your e-mail address or the profile you've submitted to the system are gender-neutral, you can expect extra scrutiny.

So feel free to engage in role-playing, as long as you're not abusing anyone's privacy. One of the most revolutionary aspects of online chat is that men and women have the opportunity to learn a great deal about each other's sexuality, whether through role-playing or—as this survey respondent indicates—through approaching each other respectfully and in a spirit of open inquiry:

> I'm about as queer as they come, and yet once I met a guy online who seemed interesting and nice. He seemed very honest, and we chatted for quite a bit, telling each other about our lives. We decided to tell each other explicit stories, which was fun for both of us. At one point I said, "Imagine this: we can teach each other what it is to be penetrated. Isn't that cool?" And he replied, "You may be a big bull dyke, but you made this heterosexual dick hard."

Taking Your Relationship into RL

Of course, the only situation in which you might truly be devastated to discover that your online Juliet is actually a Romeo or vice versa is if you've harbored hopes for an offline rendezvous. Many people do make the transition from chatting online to meeting face-to-face, but as they say on the Internet, "your mileage may vary." Perhaps you'll become friends, perhaps lovers, perhaps life partners—or perhaps you'll never want to meet again. The only thing predictable about an RL meeting is its unpredictability, but you'll minimize your chances of disappointing—or potentially dangerous—situations if you keep the following words of caution in mind.

If you and your cyberpal have agreed you'd like to meet, arrange an opportunity to speak on the phone first, as this will allow you to get a better sense of each other. Some Web sites offer a fee-based service allowing both of you to call a centralized system that connects you via an anonymous phone call—this way, you needn't give out your phone number until you're completely comfortable doing so. You may want to exchange photos ahead of time, but of course, there's no guarantee that the person you meet will resemble his or her photo.

Arrange to meet in a public place, and make sure that a friend knows where you'll be. It's a good idea to contact this friend at a prearranged time during or after your date to confirm that you're okay. We've all heard stories of people who have traveled across the country to meet an online flame. If you're going to do this, you should take extra precautions: make sure you have your own place to stay and enough money to get home safely.

Don't assume that you'll have sex face-to-face just because you've shared erotic fantasies online. You may find you don't hit it off, aren't physically

WHAT
WOMEN WANT

"The best sex, obviously, is with someone literate enough to "paint a picture" describing activities or thoughts. I suppose that in face-to-face activities, someone stupid could still be extraordinarily sexy. But stupid doesn't work online, at least not for me."

attracted to each other, or just aren't interested. More important, if you're not expecting to have sex, you're less likely to feel pressured into doing anything you don't want to. There's always the chance that you might become friends, rather than lovers.

Then again, you might wind up having great sex and leave it at that. One survey respondent told us, "When I met an online date in person, we had perhaps the best real sex I'd ever experienced. He isn't someone I'd fall in love with, or even someone I'm likely to date seriously. Still, the experience was quite positive." As sex educators, we feel compelled to remind you to be prepared—don't leave home without safer-sex supplies.

It's easy to build high expectations of an RL meeting, since you've probably developed a much greater level of intimacy in your cyber-relationship than you're used to achieving with an offline date. However, there are no guarantees that this sense of intimacy will survive the reality of a face-to-face encounter. We're not suggesting that these online relationships are somehow illusory or not *real*, but they aren't necessarily going to provide you with all you're looking for in a real-life relationship. As one survey respondent notes, "Ours was a relationship in every way, except that it was removed from the physical plane. I won't call it 'virtual,' because we both existed and exchanged real information, feelings, and expressions of love. Unfortunately, when we met, the physical attraction was just not there." You might experience this same physical letdown, or you might find that you simply don't connect in person with the intensity that you did in writing.

And, just to state the obvious, you should by no means break up with your partner, quit your job, or move to another state for the sake of a cyberlover, unless you have had numerous face-to-face meetings and both of you have seriously considered all the ramifications. Sure, lightning can strike—the two of you may turn your lives upside-down and then live happily ever after. On the other hand, you might live to regret it. As one sage survey respondent notes, "I've seen people get emotionally devastated—really, really destroyed by falling in love with an impossible person. It never seems to be equal: one person is just fooling around, while the other is hopelessly in love. It's not a good hobby for unstable people."

Some people have found their true loves in chat rooms, but sex-specific chat rooms usually cater to those in need of more immediate gratification. More often, people who fall in love online do so in the context of getting to know each other through a common interest such as a writing group, a professional organization, or a discussion group related to a particular hobby. Sometimes this common interest can have a sexual component—such as discussing BDSM or writing erotic fan fiction—but the relationship, and any accompanying cybersex, usually evolves out of an initial emotional connection.

What's the Appeal of Cybersex?

At this point, we'll step aside and yield control of the floor to our enthusiastic survey respondents—women of all ages who describe the many ways in which cybersex has enhanced their self-confidence and their sex lives.

You Aren't Limited—Or Judged—by Physical Appearances

I learned that when appearance doesn't enter into it, there is a world of potentially compatible partners, of all different (legal) ages. We are such a suppressed society; online sex is a wonderful invention. Now, if only everyone could type faster!

I am fat, and few people in real life would be attracted to me, but online it becomes irrelevant (though I am honest with my partners about it). I prefer not to see pictures of my online partners, either. Online chat gives me an opportunity to practice my ideals of honoring the mind and soul, not the body. Online, sex becomes wrapped up in verbal sparring and delving deeper into each other's brains than is usually possible in RL. In fact, much of the time, actual sexual activity and coming are secondary—the discussion, the being turned on, the mental foreplay is what it's all about. When you meet someone who is like-minded, it's like having your favorite erotic book come alive and become tailored to you personally.

Online, I find myself to be more open and more comfortable with talking about my out-of-the-ordinary fantasies and ideas. Perhaps it's because no real eye contact is involved, and therefore I don't have to worry about how the other person is reacting to what I'm expressing. Cybersex has helped me find parts of myself that I never knew existed.

You Can Explore Any Fantasy in Complete Safety

Just as in personal fantasy, you don't have to worry about mechanics—your legs stretch as wide open as you wish, there are no unseemly smells or tastes or textures, and your partner looks precisely as good as you want him or her to look.

Many of us are voyeurs who've never acted on it. With a creative partner and a little imagination, we can all become voyeurs online, picturing the images that the other person shares with us. Online there is no rejection based on appearance, no bad hair days, no disease, no regrets in the morning.

Chat gives me the opportunity to be sexual with people I could never be sexual with in real life. I'm married and monogamous, so I cannot and will not have sex with others physically; however, online I can have sex without guilt or pretense. My spouse is aware and approves and does the same himself. We consider it a healthy pressure valve for monogamy and we are brutally honest with our online partners about our unavailability in RL.

I think the appeal of cybersex is most powerful for people who are verbal and have a vivid imagination. There are no limits physically or romantically. My favorite memory of a cybersex experience was when my then-partner described a special evening for us: he toasted me with a bottle of champagne from my birth year, took me to the top of a hotel where a helicopter (similar to the president's) was waiting to take us for an evening flight, and—while listening to Pink Floyd's "Dark Side of the Moon"—we flew into space and around the moon. Now *that* couldn't have happened anywhere but the cyberworld!

Through the "magic" of cybersex, you can tear expensive clothes without spending a cent; you can put yourself in a castle tower, a dungeon, or a city on another planet; you can be any age, gender, description, or species; you can be as strong or weak as you want; children can experiment without fear; adults can be young; the wheelchair-bound can walk; and you can acquire all sorts of horribly costly equipment simply by saying "I have this." It's like being an anatomically correct Looney Toon.

Online erotic experiences have helped me figure out what I want, much as reading erotica has. I've also gotten the sense of "sampling the population" that most teenagers get by sleeping or dating around in RL, without risking disease, pregnancy, or people stalking me after we've broken up. For me, online encounters are most often about experiencing something new. I've been able to do things that are illegal or "immoral"—threesomes, foursomes, simulated bestiality (with a mythical beast!), statutory rape from both sides—without fear of legal repercussions.

Cybersex appeals to the writer in me. It allows me to be any character that I choose, to perform any fantasy, to cut loose and be as creative as I want. It doesn't have the intimacy of phone sex with a friend. Instead, cybersex always has a note of playfulness.

I love chat, whether it is focused on sex or not. Most people open up online because of the anonymity, and they can "try on" different aspects of their sensual personality. I like to think of it as a bit like playing dress-up: you have to try things on in order to find out what you like and don't like. Then you can let go of the things that don't suit you, and enhance the things that do. It's a safe way to try out sexual attitudes and behaviors.

You Can Nurture a Long-Distance Relationship

Being online has saved my long-distance relationship, which continued to grow because online we were able to talk, tell each other intimate things, have sex, express our love, have arguments, and work through them. After only one year, I can truly say I have more intimacy with my current lover than I have ever had with anyone in my life.

My lover and I do a lot of cybersex because, at present, we live two thousand miles apart. It helps us maintain our closeness and keeps fresh our memories of past intimacies until we see each other again.

You Can Learn New Things About Yourself

My whole sexuality has changed since I got online. I discovered that I'm bisexual and submissive. Before the computer, I didn't know anything about either of those parts of me.

As a result of my online experiences, my whole life has changed! It's been very freeing and therapeutic for me. After ten years of going through therapy for several abuse issues from my childhood, I've been able to open up to my friends online. Also after eighteen years of being married and functioning only as a heterosexual female (even though I did have one female lover before I was married), I was finally able to safely explore my lesbian side online, to the point where I'm now a practicing bisexual in my RL. Being able to talk about intimate sexual issues with my online friends and hearing their viewpoints and experiences has helped me make some hard choices in RL and has given me more perspective on my life and my sexual practices.

The openness of my conversations with others, both men and women, has enhanced my personal sex life and given me the impetus to shed some of my staunch New England inhibitions. My husband has no complaints about that.

One thing I've learned about virtual sex is something I think might be a difference in emphasis for men and women. I take time to set the stage and the mood before moving to the actual lovemaking. My lover doesn't linger too long on establishing a scenario, but he does a fantastic job of describing the interplay of all the senses—touching, smelling, seeing, hearing, tasting. This man, who has never seen or touched me, knows my body and its responses better than either of my two former husbands.

My online experiences have been very liberating and have made me a bit more adventurous and outspoken in the real world. I grew up in a very strict religious home and I have had to overcome a lot of backward thinking about women and sex. Online, I've been able to experiment with different fantasies in a safe environment.

My online experiences have helped me discover many things about my own sexuality and have given me the freedom to think and speak uninhibitedly. My real-world interactions have expanded to reflect this new freedom. Interestingly, one of the things I'm often told by men I meet both online and in real life is that I'm more open and honest about discussing sexual matters than anyone they've met before. By this, I don't mean cybersex or phone sex—I mean just talking about sex: about what works, doesn't work, feels good, doesn't feel good. Now I can talk about my experiences and desires in a matter-of-fact way.

I was in a relationship where there was no sex and I was suppressing myself sexually. Finding online sex made me relax the part of myself that I had been holding back both sexually and emotionally. It eventually helped me leave a nine-year relationship.

Good grief—my sex life has improved tenfold! Probably because now I think about sex so much. My own personal theory is that the more you think about sex, the more you want it, because thinking about it gets you in the mood. Supposedly, men think about sex something like six times an hour. If we women thought about it that much, we might be more interested, too. In fact, these days I am the aggressor more often than my husband. He is a happy man since I discovered cybersex.

But, It May Not Be for You

The nature of chat means, to me, that communication won't ever be as deep as face-to-face communication. I don't think you should have any illusions that what you're doing is anything more than conversing with someone from the safety and privacy of your own home, without even the level of intimacy that hearing another person's voice affords.

I am often the most lonely after I've spent a day talking to people on the computer. I don't think I'm alone in feeling that way.

What's Next?

The most intriguing aspect of chat is that, so far, it has been almost entirely text-based. People are connecting with one another purely through the power of words, and in the process they are transcending great distances, social divides, and all the assumptions that we make—based on accents, physical mannerisms, and appearances—when we meet face to face. Many people relish the liberating anonymity of online communication, so it should come as no surprise that even when there's an option to exchange or post photos—in chat rooms or on personals boards—the majority of users opt to remain invisible.

But technological advances may be changing all that. After all, the text-based nature of chat has been a product of technological limitations: slow modems result in slow transmission of photos and videos, and simple text provides the greatest immediate gratification. As bandwidth (a measurement related to the speed of data transmission over an online connection) increases and PC-compatible video technology gets both more sophisticated and more affordable, the same Joes and Janes who are crowding into chat rooms are going to have access to a whole new bag of tricks.

Many of our survey respondents compared chat to phone sex, and it won't be long before sound transmission on the Web improves so much that it will be possible to audio-chat anonymously, rather than typing back and forth. One hot new communications product is the Internet screenphone, designed to provide easy access to the Web—with this kind of technology, visually enhanced phone-sex sessions cannot be far behind.

Anyone who has ever tuned in to the jerky, almost strobelike images of streaming video on the Web is painfully aware that real-time interactive video technology is still in its infancy. But operators of and subscribers to adult pay sites aren't the only ones breathlessly awaiting technological improvements—plenty of nonprofessionals are already performing for other consenting adults online, and their numbers are bound to increase as the speed and quality of video transmission increases. Every new communications medium of the past few decades has stimulated the creation of a more democratic range of sexual materials. Once upon a time, desktop publishing brought a diverse group of erotica writers out of the closet. At about the same time, the video camcorder inspired enthusiastic amateur performers to produce their own homemade porn. Now, creative individuals across the country are employing video conferencing as the latest high-tech sex toy.

Video conferencing—in which digital cameras allow video images to be transmitted back and forth over the Internet—was developed as a business tool, but numerous satisfied voyeurs and exhibitionists around the country can testify that it has some interesting possibilities outside the office. The software known as "CU-SeeMe" (by now you should be able to translate this cutesy Web-speak for "see you, see me") allows users to connect visually either one-on-one or in anonymous group conferences. You can receive someone else's video images without having a camera yourself, but to send images, you'll need either a video capture board and camcorder or a digital camera (QuickCams are quite cheap). Once you're up and running, you can perform on each other's computer screens simultaneously and communicate either via a text-based chat window or with the software's audio component. Fans of CU-SeeMe hook up with each other through switchboardlike servers called "reflectors" or through listings on IRC channels such as #Cuseemesex. See the "Real-Time Resources" listings (p. 177) for links to relevant software and hardware sites. As the following survey respondents indicate, CU-SeeMe has its fans, but it isn't to everyone's taste.

I've only experienced CU-SeeMe once. I watched a friend masturbate, and thought that was kind of silly. But, the idea of being able to see the person you're talking to is pretty spectacular.

I really don't want to be on display on someone's computer screen. An exhibitionist I am not . . . though I would watch.

I loved being on CU-See Me. It's flattering to have people gawking at you. And you know you're giving a good show if everyone else stops typing.

We would venture to guess that no matter what technological advancements come along, many people will continue to employ text-based chat in getting to know online friends and lovers. It will be a matter of personal taste whether they decide to amplify their online experiences with sound and visuals. Certainly, some folks will be delighted to add the enhancement of audio and video to their repertoire—whether in order to explore fantasies with other consenting partners or to spice up a long-distance romance. Others, like this survey respondent, will prefer to stick with words:

I think as computers and phone lines evolve to faster and faster transfer protocols, video conferencing might be worth using one day. But I'll be sad if we move in that direction universally. The fascinating thing about the Internet to me is that we have truly left our prejudices behind. Color, age, gender, disability, apparent class—none of these things make any difference. For the first time, people are connecting solely on the basis of what they have to say, and what's in their minds. I find this utterly compelling, and I would love to see it run its course.

In any event, as we noted at the beginning of this chapter, technology is simply a tool and a toy. It can't change you—though you may change yourself as a result of what you've learned through your explorations. While online communication has given many women new information about their own fantasies, desires, and sexuality, it still takes as much courage to put this self-knowledge into practice offline as it ever has. And there is still plenty of room for improvement in the resources available to women in real life. As Heartless of Heartless's Holey Haven (see p. 88) comments dryly, "It doesn't matter what kind of technological advances are made if women still aren't having their sexual needs met. It's irrelevant how fast your modem is if you're still not able to find an erotic video that's been made with your tastes in mind." If online communication about sex has any single transformative effect, we hope it will be to encourage all women to overcome whatever lingering fear, shame, and embarrassment might prevent them from naming and demanding the sexual satisfaction that is their birthright.

Reviews

GENERAL RESOURCES

Art and Love on the Net

http://www.pacific-pages.com/aln

The editors of this attractive monthly e-zine state their goal is "to provide solace and support for those who are confused or uneasy about the often overwhelming onrush of emotions arising from Internet relationships." Readers submit their own art, romantic stories, poetry, and love letters. The staff of four editors (both male and female) write most of the essays and editorials, with topics such as "How the Internet is changing our perceptions of gender and marriage by breaking down the socially-enforced barriers against intimate conversation between married strangers of opposite gender." When you're done with the critical analysis, you can surf over to the site's advice column, active message board, and personals to watch cyber-romantics in action. Includes annotated links to other cyber-romance and cybersex sites.

Cyber Romance 101

http://web2.airmail.net/walraven/romance.htm

Rain Walraven designed this "little pool of cyberspace" as a labor of love, in order to provide an evenhanded introduction to the subject of Internet relationships. You'll find a collection of essays and articles by psychologists, journalists, and netizens, along with book reviews, erotic fiction, links to advice columns, and links to matchmaking sites. The effect is like being handed a file folder of clippings compiled by a well-read, nonjudgmental friend. While the cyber-romance section of the site is not frequently updated, it's worth at least one visit—and you may find yourself returning more often to check out Rain's journal, poems, stories, and photos of her young son.

Cybersociology

http://www.socio.demon.co.uk/magazine/magazine.html

"A forum for the discussion of the social scientific study of cyberspace," *Cybersociology* is a sporadically published magazine devoted to the topics of cyberspace, the Internet, and online communities. Articles, book reviews, and site reviews by both academics and lay people are admirably well written and interesting. The first issue of this e-zine was devoted to cybersex; for more on the same topic, check out editor Robin Hamman's masters thesis about cybersex and AOL, found at http://www.socio.demon.co.uk/Cyborgasms.html.

Life on the Internet: Netiquette

http://www.screen.com/start/guide/netiquette.html

This excellent gateway site links to book excerpts and articles about netiquette, including Charles Hymes's tips for spotting Internet hoaxes, the "Unofficial Smiley Dictionary," a guide to acronyms, and the tongue-in-cheek teachings of Emily Postnews.

Connectix

http://www.connectix.com

The manufacturers of the QuickCam digital camera provide detailed product information on their site, along with tips on how to use the QuickCam for video conferencing and how to set up your own webcam site.

Hotmail Free, Anonymous E-Mail

http://www.hotmail.com

This free, anonymous, web-based e-mail service is sponsored by Microsoft.

ICQ Software

http://www.mirabilis.com

Download free ICQ software from this site.

Internet Relay Chat Help

http://www.irchelp.org

An excellent introduction to the wide world of Internet Relay Chat (IRC), this site includes a FAQ section, manuals, links to software downloads, channel listings, and more. A spin-off of the help archive from EFnet, one of the largest IRC networks, the site also links to information from other sources.

IRC-Related Documents

http://urth.acsu.buffalo.edu/irc/WWW/ircdocs.html

This directory of IRC-related Web resources is not completely up to date, so a number of the links provided are defunct. However, the site is so rich in links and listings that you're bound to find useful information here. Plus, it's not affiliated with a particular IRC network, so it has a nice "nondenominational" feel.

The MUD Resource Collection

http://www.godlike.com/muds

A thorough list of links to MUD-related resources, including FAQs, articles, and lists of client software and host servers.

White Pine

http://www.wpine.com/Products/CU-SeeMe

White Pine manufactures the premiere video-conferencing software, CU-SeeMe, and while their site emphasizes the software's use in business and technology (see how NASA puts CU-SeeMe to work!), you'll also find a directory of public video chat sites, where you should be able to get access to information on less technical uses. You can download a demo copy of the software for free.

Yahoo!

http://www.yahoo.com/recreation/games/internet_games

Listings for MUDs, MUSHes, MOOS, etc.

CHATS AND CONFERENCES

Isadora Alman's Sexuality Forum

http://www.askisadora.com

Justly famed for her humorous, no-nonsense, nationally syndicated sex advice column, Isadora Alman has led a loyal band of fans into cyberspace. Her Web site includes a searchable database of past "Ask Isadora" Q&A columns, online ordering of her books and audiotapes, a chat room, and a bustling public conference that attracts hundreds of daily postings from all around the country. Isadora makes occasional posts to her conference, but by and large, this friendly community is self-moderated by a gang of thoughtful and curious posters. Topics range all over the map, from rimming to romance. There's no fee, but you must register with the site's management, which reserves the right to boot the discourteous.

Bianca's Smut Shack

http://www.bianca.com

Ah, Bianca. This imaginary creature is the loving, semidivine hostess who presides over a gloriously disorganized online community comprised of "Shacks," each devoted to a different general topic: art, hobbies, technology, culture . . . and, of course, sex. Bianca has been spreading the mantra of sex-positivity in her legendary Smut Shack since the Web's Ice Age—1994, that is. The "trolls" who administer this site adopt an attitude of benign neglect, and content and tone are controlled by the hordes of visitors who pour through the bedroom, bathroom, closet, and other virtual rooms of Bianca's Smut Shack every day.

If some of the rooms are too raunchy for your taste, check around—with members adding their own chat areas and forums all the time, you're sure to find a congenial space somewhere in the Shack (or you can always mosey over to the Kitchen's "Ramen Romper Room" for a discussion of this magical

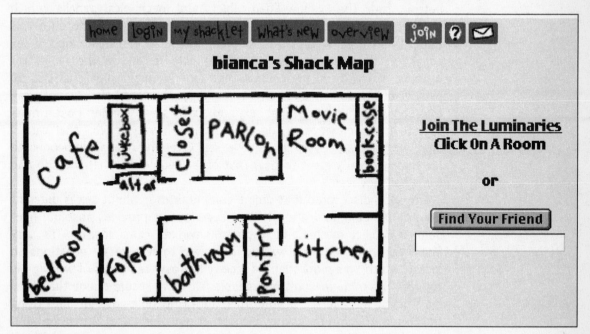

food). The site's conferences and real-time chat are easy to use, and Bianca cheerfully notes that if you get "tired of the jerks and impostors" you may find in the public chat rooms, you can always pay a small annual fee for the privilege of access to private chat. Bianca also offers a phone-chat service, so you can talk to your fellow "Biancanauts" on either a group party-line or a one-on-one date line without giving out your home phone number.

Profile: Isadora
Alman

Isadora Alman's
Sexuality Forum

http://www.
askisadora.com

For over ten years, Isadora Alman has been dispensing eminently sensible advice on sex and relationships via her Q&A column, "Ask Isadora," which is syndicated to alternative weeklies from the *Village Voice* to the *San Francisco Bay Guardian*. Humorous, yet never flip; straight-shooting, yet never disrespectful—Isadora delivers tips on meeting, mating, and communication that have won her legions of loyal fans. Therefore, when first approached about taking her show online, she assumed that her Web site would be more business as usual: that visitors to her site would provide the questions and she would provide the answers. But as the conference and chat environment of "Isadora Alman's Sexuality Forum" evolved, she discovered that online, by definition, there is no absolute authority—everyone's an expert!

A self-professed technophobe who had to be "dragged kicking and screaming into the twenty-first century," Isadora was coaxed into putting aside the "yellow-lined tablets and mechanical pencils, which had been writing requirements for most of my life, to come onto this thing. What I really wanted to do was provide an immediate kind of sex education that hitherto I'd only been able to do on the radio. For instance, if I write in my column that some women enjoy anal sex, 50 percent of my audience is going to think 'yeah, right.' However, if I say that some women enjoy anal sex, and six or seven women post a message to the conference saying, 'yes, I enjoy it very much,' that carries more weight than anything I can ever say. Over and over again people tell me that it's really great to hear that other people do what they do and feel what they feel."

She soon discovered that online communication about sex is different from offline communication in two key ways: it provides absolute freedom of subject matter and inspires immediate camaraderie. "The very first week that the Forum was up, I received three separate questions on incest, which was more than I'd received in over ten years of writing my column. For some reason these people felt more secure online than they did sending me a letter. Beyond this, a lot of people got right into using the Forum *as* a forum, asking each other questions like 'Where on your body do you like to be kissed? What's your favorite sexual position?'

Really, they just wanted to get information from other people that they could not get in their own life. And that they could not get from a single respondent, like me."

In fact, to a certain extent Isadora's online experience is that of being "rendered superfluous. After all, if some guy says, 'I want to know how to go down on my wife,' forty-seven people are ready and willing to tell him. While I'd love it if therapists were made obsolete because everybody had a happy life, I do feel kind of unneeded online." Of course, this society has a long way to go before sex advisors are rendered obsolete. Isadora notes that "At least twice a week, we'll get the question, Is my penis big enough? Or, do men like such and such? These are the questions that I've answered a gazillion times, to which the only answer is that there *is* no general rule and that people differ and so forth—well, if I've given the answer yesterday, a new poster will come in with the same question today."

Forum users are able to talk intimately about everything from relationships to technique, and Isadora compares the sense of connection experienced by regular users of her forum with that of consciousness-raising groups of the '70s. She views the interactions among women and men on the Forum as a training ground for improving communication offline: "This same kind of community that they see online, wherein they can talk about their most private fears and desires, is perfectly possible in real life. It just takes a little work." If you want to practice your own communication skills in a low-risk environment, and pick up a few new sex tips to boot, there's a place at the conference table waiting for you.

Profile: Isadora Alman, continued

Dalnet BDSM Channel for Adults

http://members.bellatlantic.net/~gwriter/bdsm.html

The homepage for the IRC channel #bdsm is a fount of information about all aspects of both IRC and BDSM. If you're new to either world, you'll particularly appreciate this friendly, welcoming site, which dishes up equal measures of technical advice and general encouragement. You'll find links to sites with IRC software, a general introduction to the rules of this particular channel, and channel logs (text from scenes that participants have given permission to quote), as well as a schedule of upcoming channel conferences and text logs from previous conferences. The channel logs provide an excellent opportunity to get familiar with the style of IRC speak. The site also includes a brief description of

BDSM, erotic stories and poems by channel regulars, articles about dominance and submission, and the opportunity to subscribe to a listserv about BDSM issues.

Deja News

http://www.dejanews.com

This Web interface to Internet discussion groups is an extraordinarily user-friendly gateway to the vast resources of over fifty thousand Usenet newsgroups, one-third of which are thoroughly archived on the site. The site's FAQs provide an excellent introduction to the wide world of Usenet. You can search the archives, browse current postings, and—once you've registered for free with the site—post your own messages: look under the "rec" hierarchy for groups such as "rec.arts.movies.erotica" or under the "soc" hierarchy for "soc.sexuality.general." Binary files—that is, graphics and photos—aren't available through Deja News, but given the wealth of fascinating reading that is available, we doubt you'll miss visual aids. The downside is that you can't post directly to moderated newsgroups through Deja News, but the upside is that all spam is filtered out of the postings you do see and you have access to a greater number of newsgroups than you would through your ISP.

Dimensions

http://www.dimensionsmagazine.com

Dimensions is the online version of a bimonthly print magazine that "explains relationships, experiences, fat sex, and sexuality from the unique perspective of BBWs and their admirers." BBWs are big, beautiful women, and this great site includes discussion boards, personal ads, and links to related "sexy and special interest" sites. The personals aren't free, but the boards and magazine content are.

A Dyke's World

http://dykesworld.de

Indina Beuche is the charming hostess of this lesbian site, which features an impressive array of sexual materials and links, as well as information on Indina's many other interests. Check out her chat room (not exclusively devoted to sex chat), free personals, and Pillowtalk discussion board—"dedicated to the lust and tragedies of sex and love and built for women-loving women." Indina also hosts the Wild Women Dreamin' Wet page of lesbian erotica (see p. 31). Since Indina is German and has traveled extensively in Africa, this is one site that truly does have an international flavor.

Grrltalk: The Guide to Lesbian Chat

http://www.grrltalk.net

Ooh, girlfriend! Have you ever fantasized about meeting a devastatingly competent butch who could show you the ropes online? Well, we've got the answer to your dreams, and her name is Muskie—the online handle of activist, writer, Web designer, and radical lesbian feminist Laura Tisoncik. Her awe-inspiring resource site features listings of every chat room and IRC channel of possible interest to lesbians, both sex-related and not. Best of all, Muskie has compiled a brilliant array of introductory articles that are a gold mine for chat novices of all sexualities: from "The Clueless Newbie's Introduction to Online Chat" to lesbian chat netiquette to tips on combating online harassment to a step-by-step guide to getting started on IRC. Muskie also hosts her own message board and chat room, and her site includes a comprehensive array of links to other chat and IRC resource sites. While this site does not offer sex-related content, it is a one-of-a-kind gateway resource to the world of online relationships.

GrrlZ on GrrlZ

http://www.womyn.org/grrlz.html

A nicely designed site offering personal ads and chat for women seeking women.

Talk City

http://www.talkcity.com

You'll find literally hundreds of chat rooms here at one of the Web's largest chat sites. Head to the "People and Connecting" channel to find chats listed under "Romance" and "Courtship Corner." Talk City also hosts moderated chats on different topics, such as cyberdating and the art of writing romance novels. And even WebTV users can access real-time chat through this site.

Thrive Online Passion

http://www.thriveonline.com/passion.html

The Thrive Passion message boards are filled with thousands of discussions on topics such as sexual health, debates on human sexuality, dating, and sexual techniques. These well-maintained boards are easy to read and use. The site also features scheduled chats hosted by Thrive's resident sexpert, Delilah, and "sex doc" Dr. Sandor Gardos as well as a "cyberlove board" called "Love Happens," offering ICQ chat, love and relationship advice, and a link to personals at Match.com.

RANT: ONLINE JARGON

You know what emoticons are, right? They're the little sideways faces that many folks sprinkle through their online communiqués—they convey emotion using icons. A smile :-) or a wink ;-) are the ones you'll see most often, usually to indicate a "just kidding" comment—so you'll also see these icons referred to as "smileys." While some of our best Web friends make lavish use of emoticons, we just don't get it. How did the online community—which is largely populated by smart, sarcastic, iconoclastic wiseacres—settle on a communications tool that looks like a Hello Kitty marketing campaign? You can't fool us—those are smiley faces! And they're not just ubiquitous, they're insidious; despite our own active disdain, we can't count the number of times our fingers have started to creep toward the colon and close-parens keys.

Emoticons evolved out of the fact that, in the absence of visual cues, written text can appear more confrontational than intended; it's not always easy to communicate that you're making a joke. Hence the smiley faces. We've got no beef with the desire to be nonconfrontational, but we're a lot more comfortable with coping mechanisms that involve words, or at least letters—after all, aren't we supposed to be writing to each other? Color us conservative, but this is not an Etch-a-Sketch we're communicating on

here. Many online regulars sidestep the emoticon issue by using shortcuts such as <g> (meaning "grin"). Okay, this is admittedly pretty cutesy too, but it still beats those sideways faces.

Similarly, if you spend any time communicating online, you'll notice certain mysterious acronyms popping up everywhere. Folks in chat rooms or on conferences are usually typing in a hurry, so they rely on a shorthand for common words ("R" for "are," "C" for "see," and "U" for "you") and common expressions, such as LOL (laughing out loud); IMHO (in my humble opinion); BTW (by the way); and so on. Of course, as with any slang, these expressions exist in large part just to separate the hip crowd of regulars from those wet behind the ears.

Many Web guidebooks reprint glossaries of emoticons and acronyms as if they were the Rosetta Stone, solemnly instructing newbies that the fastest way to feel at home and be accepted online is to adopt their use. We're not about to go that far. After all—like your mom told you in high school—we think you're swell just the way you are. But in the spirit of full disclosure, we refer the curious to a great resource site, Life on the Internet: Netiquette (p.176), which links to several extensive glossaries of emoticons and acronyms. Now, don't let anyone tell you we didn't teach you the secret handshake!

WELL (Whole Earth 'Lectronic Links)

http://www.well.com

Before the Web, online communities took shape in bulletin boards (BBSs), members-only forums in which groups of local users dialed into one centralized computer server. Probably the most famous—and infamous—BBS to go global is the San Francisco Bay Area's WELL, which *Wired* magazine dubbed "the world's most influential online community." While many old-timers would argue that the WELL's glory days are over, it still maintains a unique community feel, thanks to a policy banning anonymity and a history of RL get-togethers among members.

For a nominal monthly fee, you can join the WELL and participate in a wide range of conferences with a host of opinionated, articulate, occasionally quite obnoxious women and men. Since every topic under the sun is covered here, there are plenty of conferences related to sex. However, don't be surprised if a discussion of good erotica sites suddenly veers off into an argument over grammar—this is a contentious crowd! The upside is you won't have to field irksome queries about the size of your breasts or whether you're horny, and you might well wind up stimulating your biggest sex organ—your brain.

Yahoo! Chat

http://chat.yahoo.com

This is a user-friendly chat room courtesy of the excellent search engine, Yahoo!, which periodically schedules chats on different sexual subjects. Check out the "Romance" category for romance and more. The service is completely free, and detailed, easy-to-understand instructions will have you up and chatting in no time. Yahoo! also provides free, anonymous e-mail, should you wish to launch a passionate correspondence.

DATING SITES

These are the more popular dating sites, most of which take ads from hopefuls of all sex styles.

Authoritative Matchmaker

http://www.awarenet.com/amm

Match.com

http://www.match.com

One and Only Internet Personals

http://www.one-and-only.com

Web Personals

http://www.webpersonals.com

Yahoo Personals

http://personals.yahoo.com

or look for sites in Yahoo, under:

http://www.yahoo.com/society_and_culture/relationships/dating

http://www.yahoo.com/business_and_economy/classifieds/personals

Chapter <u>Eight</u>

Directories, Search Engines, and Links

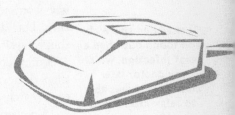

You may have started this book convinced that the Web doesn't have much to offer women in the way of sexual materials. Now that you're near the end, perhaps the realization that your cup runneth over has left you feeling a little overwhelmed. Never fear—there are plenty of ways to seize control of the seemingly infinite amounts of sex information and entertainment that await your gaze!

At some point, you'll want to venture beyond the sites listed in this book. Hundreds of new Web sites are posted every day, and old sites frequently change their addresses. Fortunately, online research tools like directories and search engines can assist you in tracking down the site or sites you seek according to key phrase, site name, or general subject. And if you're looking for new material suited to your tastes, one of your favorite site's list of hand-picked links can be your best source of up-to-date, quality leads.

Search Engines

Your browser includes a "Net Search" function, which sends you to any one of several sites (such as Alta Vista, Webcrawler, or Lycos) known as search engines. Search engines sift through the Web's labyrinth of pages and retrieve data based on specific key words that you designate. For example, when you type in the phrase "female+condom," you'll end up with a list of links to sites that contain those words. Commands that will help you refine your search are explained on each search engine's site. The "+" in this example tells the search engine to retrieve only sites in which the words *female* and *condom* appear together; otherwise, you would end up with thousands of listings for sites that refer to *either* female or condom. In order to narrow your search as much as possible, it's important that you choose your key words carefully. "Adult+sexuality" will call up mostly sex education sites, but "adult+sex" will call up a mixture of "hot and nasty" pay sites, shopping sites, and the occasional informational site.

Search engines are ever evolving, as companies work on ways to expand their retrieval rates, reduce the number of links to obsolete sites, and fine-tune search results. At present, search engines are estimated to cover as little as 15 percent of the material on the Web, and different engines perform better in different subject areas—your best bet is not to rely on any one engine but to experiment with several.

You may have noticed that we refer to a "search function" in many of our site reviews. Individual sites use this tool, which operates on the same keyword principle as search engines, to help visitors locate specific information within the site. Sites with many pages and large archives are routinely incorporating search functions.

Directories

Many search engines also provide directories, where sites are manually categorized by subject matter, much as in a card catalog or the Yellow Pages. You start your quest with primary category headings, which branch out into seemingly infinite subcategories. Unfortunately, none of the general directories—including the most popular consumer directory, Yahoo!—include sex as a main category heading (despite the fact that *sex* is the word most frequently used in searches), so you need to do a little detective work to deduce where the sex sites might be categorized (you may have had a comparable experience looking for sex books in a bookstore!). For instance, sex toy stores are usually listed under "Businesses," safer sex under "Health," and erotica under "Entertainment." Once you do unearth your area of interest, directories are ideal for locating abundant site listings within very specific categories. Each directory features its own set of bells and whistles—some provide cross-referencing, some offer news and chat, some let you customize your own page of links.

A large directory will often list purely factual, one-line descriptions of sites, but consumer-friendly directories, such as Jane's Net Sex Guide and Eroscan, provide detailed descriptions and opinionated reviews. Use these especially when you want to "look before you leap" into an unknown site.

When visiting adult directories, or when searching using sexually explicit words, be prepared for a barrage of explicit adult banner ads. Even "tasteful" sites need to pay their staff, and advertising is a key source of revenue.

Link Pages

Some individual sites feature detailed lists of links that reflect the author's specific interests. We've included several such sites here, since they provide an excellent gateway to resources that we were unable to cover fully in this book. In general, link sites are maintained as an individual labor of love, so you won't find the preponderance of ad banners that characterize the adult directories.

Individual sites are increasingly banding together in "Web rings" such as the "Sex Education Web Ring" or the "Banned Sites Web Ring." A Web ring links participating sites with a logo or text link at the bottom of each site's homepage. You can travel on a circular path among all the linked sites and end up back at your original destination. Web rings have a slightly cliquish aspect, but they provide a way for individual sites to actively endorse one another and for surfers to discover a group of philosophically similar sites—sort of like having a bookstore clerk whose opinion you respect recommend all her favorite books.

By using a combination of the tools just described, you should be able to find sites that answer all your questions and scratch all your itches. And if you need a final reminder of the value of search tools, try this one on for size: the last time we searched using just the word *sex*, we received 1,376,149 listings. Now you know a few ways to look for that needle in the haystack!

Reviews

Ann Rose's Ultimate Birth Control Links

http://gynpages.com/ultimate

A gold mine of practical information, this painstakingly thorough set of links covers traditional contraceptive methods such as the pill, IUD, and condoms as well as birth control options such as homosexuality and alternatives to intercourse. A family planning counselor for twenty years, Ann states her opinions freely and with humor. Her heading for the rhythm method section reads, "I got rhythm, oops, I got pregnant," and she arranges photos of various well-known male conservatives (the pope, Newt Gingrich, and Rush Limbaugh) under the heading "Who you should not listen to about birth control."

Bisexual Internet Resources

http://www.bisexual.org/BiResources.html

A comprehensive list of Web resources specifically created for bisexual women and men. Includes organizational sites, individual Web pages, information on bi-related books sold online, and IRC channels, mailing lists, and newsgroups with bi content. These links are part of the Bisexual Options site, some of which is maintained in cooperation with the international site bi.org.

Complete Internet Sex Resources Guide (CISRG)

http://www.sleepingbeauty.com/world/netsex.html

This directory of mainstream adult Web sites also lists newsgroups, mailing lists, FTP sites, and gopher sites related to sex.

Ds Kiosk: A Power Exchange Resource Center

http://www.cuffs.com/link-filter.htm

This exceptional "links library" categorizes approximately three thousand Web pages related to all aspects of BDSM and fetish sexuality, with an emphasis on online encounters. The links are one part of an excellent resource site designed by maledom "Artful" and his femsub "natasha" specifically "as a resource for the online community involved in DS (Dominant & submissive) relationships," as well as a forum for exploring the emotions and experiences of their own online relationship. You'll find a wealth of erotica, information, and discussion boards on this excellent gateway site.

Eroscan Index: The Index of the Adult Internet

http://www.eroscan.com

This directory goes for quality as well as quantity by combining extensive listings of commercial, informational, and alternative sites with a number of consumer-friendly functions. All listings include brief descriptions, but many sites are also reviewed in more detail. An annotated table of contents will help you find the categories you're interested in, but the multitude of cross-referenced subcategories gets a little confusing. The site map is useful for quick reference, though it is so extensive it can load slowly, which defeats the purpose. A search function, a key to help identify content quickly, and a FAQ section also assist viewers. Expect an abundance of adult banner ads.

Female Ejaculation and G-Spot Links

http://w1.240.telia.com/~u24000041

A unique collection of links to pictures, articles, videos, stories, FAQs, interviews, and discussions of female ejaculation and the G-spot.

Gender Issues

http://drycas.club.cc.cmu.edu/~julie/gender.html

Julie, a bisexual feminist, offers a superior collection of links related to transgender issues, covering commercial, informational, and regional resources as well as online discussion groups and personal homepages. She supplements her links with a gallery of gender images and spotlights offbeat articles and sites. We enjoyed her personal statement: "I've come to view humanity as more of a smorgasbord of gender and sexuality than two doors, one marked 'men' and another marked 'women.' We create our own gender, through our own choices. Some people have changed gender by climbing over the walls that exist. As far as I'm concerned we can only be free by tearing down the walls that hold us into a fixed and rigid construct of what it means to be ourselves."

Jane's Net Sex Guide

http://www.janesguide.com

After wasting too much time visiting adult sites that didn't live up to their hype, Jane and her partner Jim decided to take on the enormous task of reviewing adult Web sites. They've compiled hundreds of site descriptions and reviews, with particularly comprehensive listings for photo sites, categorized according to sexual orientations and activities. You'll also find recommendations for adult shopping sites, phone sex lines, escort services, personals, and sex resort listings. Frank and opinionated, Jane takes a democratic approach to her selection—reviewing plenty of queer-friendly and women's sites along with more conventional adult sites. Her reviews are particularly hilarious when she takes aim at sites with too much advertising and those running scams designed to part users with their money. An advocate for adult consumers online, Jane offers consumer tips, investigates complaints, and features a "Hall of Shame" for the most obnoxious offenders—her site is a must-read for anyone thinking of subscribing to pay sites. All this plus profiles and interviews with interesting online personalities add up to a site that should be a regular destination in your online travels. Because of Jane's extensive categorization, the site would be greatly enhanced with a search function. What Jane's site lacks in graphics, she makes up for with her colorful descriptions!

Kinky Flavors

http://www.kinkyflavors.com

Mistress Blanca and Peter, active members of a variety of sex-related newsgroups and authors of the now-lapsed "Pointer to Sex Info on the Net," have thoughtfully posted a series of comprehensive Resource Guides on several different themes. Each guide includes links to related Web sites as well as a summary of references from newsgroups, IRC channels, books, and print media. Here, conveniently combined on one site for your delectation, are the Masturbation Resources Guide; the Spanking Resources Guide; the Fetish Resources Guide; the FemDom Resources Guide; and the BDSM Resources Guide. All are quite up to date. Don't miss the couple's unique research and literature guide "The Dominatrix in Print and Other Media," an annotated bibliography and detailed subject index about the "Sexually Dominant Woman and Her Devotees."

The Mining Company

http://sexuality.miningco.com/mlibrary.htm

For a manageably sized, tastefully presented list of links, check out the sexuality section at The Mining Company, a directory of listings hand-picked and described by the company's "guides." The alternative adult sites in this short yet representative selection are grouped under categories such as gay and lesbian, information, sexual activities, religion, censorship, professional organizations, art, and humor. Includes a search function.

Naughty Linx

http://www.naughty.com

Once you get past the array of explicit banner ads, you'll find an extensive, well-categorized set of adult links (more mainstream than alternative), along with a search function.

The Official Site of rec.arts.movies.erotica

http://www.rame.net

If you're a fan of adult videos, have we got a resource for you. This labor of love by members of the Usenet newsgroup rec.arts.movies.erotica (the moderated successor to alt.sex.movies) serves as a gateway to the many FAQs, lists, and databases lovingly compiled by diligent r.a.m.e. regulars such as Peter van Aarle (the "Dutch Master") and Ron Wilhelm (the "Heretic"). You'll find the Adult Movie FAQ, featuring information about the adult video industry, performers, print resources, and trivia; the Adult Movie Review Index, a master index of noncommercial reviews; the RAME Reading Room, containing archived postings and interviews; and the Internet Adult Film Database, with search functions to call up information on over twelve thousand titles. Don't miss the "Adult Movie Related Links," which steers you to such valuable lists as the "Natural Busum Alliance" (celebrating silicone-free stars) and "Web Sites Devoted to Porn Stars" (both free and commercial sites). These articulate, irreverent, discriminating fans provide valuable guidance as you pan for gold in the river of cheesy porn.

"Consumers have a right to protection, whether they're buying something as mundane as a toaster or as controversial as access to porn."

Those fighting words are from Jane Duvall, the Ralph Nader of online adult commerce. As the creator of Jane's Net Sex Guide, she champions consumers' rights by offering advice on how to avoid getting ripped off, exposing fraudulent business practices, and investigating individual complaints against adult companies. She takes a full-service approach to her site, which contains categorized, annotated listings of thousands of adult sites, "from highbrow erotica to unabashed porn."

Jane and her partner Jim visit a thousand sites each month and review the best two hundred. They don't base their judgments of the sites on artistic merit or subject matter, since that, says Jane, "is a matter of taste. We look for honesty. Does a site have advertising that attempts to mislead viewers? Does a site have a preview that promises much more than the inside delivers? Is a site so full of ads that you can't find the actual content? Any of those things will get a site a bad review." In order to get a positive review, sites need to be up-front about content and pricing. Jane also notes that originality earns high marks, since most adult content online is fairly generic.

Jane's role as consumer advocate evolved out of her experience as a reviewer, which immersed her in the Web's world of adult commerce. "When I started, I was a Pollyanna of sorts, not really realizing how many rip-offs there were in the adult world," says Jane. "Were it not for all the reviewing Jim and I do, we wouldn't see what is going on." She's dedicated to giving consumers, who spend much less time online than she does, the benefit of her perspective.

Asked what piece of advice she'd most like to impart to our readers, she replied, "There has been a lot of press about the security of credit card transactions on the Internet. The real hazard, though, is making sure you are sending your card to a reputable business." She offers these pointers: Make sure the company provides a telephone number, try to verify their address, and see if you can get references. "Don't think that from the look of the site, you can tell if someone is honest or not—you can't," says Jane. (For more consumer tips, see "Shopping Tips" on p. 128 and "Savvy Subscriber Tips" on p. 63.)

If one woman taking on the online adult industry sounds a bit like David battling Goliath, it is—and Jane's slingshot gets results. Several sites have cleaned up their acts based on Jane's reviews, and educated consumers are starting to demand better service and greater accountability. Jane's site now features a "Customer Service Approved" listing of pay sites, which includes only those that adhere to a strict set of customer-service guidelines. "It is our hope that accountability will prod more sites into working on the issue of building consumer confidence," explains Jane. "Sort of a Better Business Bureau model, but for the adult Web."

Where does such a fearless leader draw her inspiration? Not surprisingly, Jane cites other strong women like Janet Reno, Hillary Clinton, and Susie Bright as role models. "But the ones who really inspire me to be vocal are people who are antisex, like the Andrea Dworkins of the world," says Jane. "I think being closed off to your sexuality creates far more social problems than pornography ever will. Once you open up inside and can deal with sexuality honestly, you're much more likely to be a happy and well-adjusted person."

Profile: Jane Duvall, continued

Prostitutes' Education Network

http://www.bayswan.org/penet.html

If you have a question related to sex work, this is the place to find answers (the site even has a helpful section for students researching the issue). You'll find links to information about prostitutes' health needs, statistics, legal issues, sex workers' rights groups, international news, educational videos, and the individual homepages of a variety of sex workers, including Margo St. James, Scarlot Harlot, and Nina Hartley.

Q World

http://www.qworld.org

This resource site for the queer community hosts message boards, chats, an informational library, links to noncommercial queer sites on the Internet, and TransWorld, an online community for transgendered people and their families and friends.

Sexhomepage

http://www.sexhomepage.com

"A resource for the study and understanding of human sexuality," Sexhomepage was designed by Judy Seifer, a sex therapist and educator, and Steven Kapelow, a producer of sex-ed videos. Reflecting their blend of professional and lay perspectives, the site's *Sex Today* e-zine features articles by therapists and educators on a variety of themes, as well as interviews with ordinary folks. The site's highlight is its ambitious "Sexuality Database," a breathtakingly comprehensive catalog of links to a huge range of sexual materials on the Web, organized by topic. From abstinence to addiction, body modification to fetishes, prostitution to romance—no topic goes unexamined. While the database draws heavily from the Web sites of the "usual suspects" (Dr. Ruth, Isadora Alman, Dr. Patti Britton, The Society for Human Sexuality, and Go Ask Alice!), it is an amazing resource for anyone who wants to look up a range of discussions on any single subject matter. The site also includes a section of commercial sex links.

Sexual Assault Information Page

http://www.cs.utk.edu/~bartley/saInfoPage.html

Thousands of links to information concerning rape, child sexual abuse and assault, incest, ritual abuse, sexual assault, and sexual harassment are provided on this nonprofit's site. Within each topic's set of links you'll find survivors' groups, online and offline crisis centers, individual homepages, and counseling services. The site has a search function and FAQ section, and a print newsletter is available for a nominal subscription fee.

Yahoo!

http://www.yahoo.com

Yahoo! is perhaps the best-known general-interest directory and search engine; its popularity might have something to do with its enormous selection of sex links. It even hosts some adult chat rooms. We only wish the folks at Yahoo would make life easier for all of us by adding a "Sex" section to the site's table of contents. As it is, you have to browse through "Health," "Business," or "Entertainment" to get to the good stuff.

Chapter Nine

Free Speech and the Future

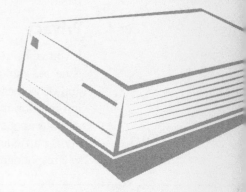

The Web has become such a hot topic in such a short amount of time that you could be excused for thinking that it's either the most amazing technological breakthrough or the most overhyped phenomenon of the century. Most likely, it's a little of both. The Web is simply a new communications tool, no more and no less. It's not about to change human nature, but it does allow individuals to make connections in ways that weren't previously possible, and to connect more easily around a topic that has been particularly absent from open discourse up until now: sexuality.

Our first book, a sex manual entitled *The New Good Vibrations Guide to Sex*, ended with a heartfelt plea to readers in which we encouraged them to take the risk of speaking up about sex. We have no way of knowing how many readers may have been inspired by that book to chat to their friends, neighbors, or family members about condom brands, adult videos, masturbation, or erotic massage. But in the several years since it was published, an entirely new medium has emerged, and individuals are entering into these very kinds of conversations and discussions with newfound online confidants. We don't expect the Web to transform the world, but we are thrilled that its accessible, anonymous, outrageous environment is bringing women and men several steps closer to the type of honest self-exploration and dialogue that is required in order for sexual pleasure to reign supreme! (That *is* our not-so-secret agenda.)

In this chapter we'll touch on a couple of the hot-button topics that are affecting how online communication will evolve, along with our hopes for the future of sexual materials on the Web.

Privacy

If you've been following the news, you're probably aware that privacy is the issue *du jour* among webmasters, service providers, government officials, and consumers alike. The Web has the potential to link such a vast array of information from such a variety of sources that consumers, in particular, are anxious about what kind of trail their surfing leaves in its wake. This anxiety is particularly acute among consumers of sexual materials, like our survey respondent who asked, "What can individuals I'm chatting with (web-

---

PRIVACY TIPS

Here are some ways to assert your rights to privacy online. For related tips on how to protect yourself from online harassment, see the "Safe Cybersex" sidebar on p. 162.

Get the facts. You have more control over how much of your personal information appears online than you're probably aware of. The first step is to find out what's out there. Try looking up your own name in search engines or online phone directories. If the listing includes information you'd prefer weren't public knowledge, you can ask the service to delete it. Did you know that it's possible for interested parties to access your ISP's registration files through a tool known as a "finger"? This is a good reason to limit the information you provide to your ISP—for instance, you might want to register as J. Doe, rather than Jane Doe. You can "finger" yourself to see what information is publicly available about your account (see the "Privacy" site listings). Most ISPs automatically block finger access, but if yours doesn't, ask that your name be removed from your finger information.

Know your cookies. A "cookie" is a piece of data about your visit to a Web site that the site stores on your computer's hard drive. Cookies track your path through a Web site and save information about your visit that can be accessed when you return to the site (for instance, distinguishing those pages you've already visited from those you haven't). Commercial companies already use cookies as part of their shopping-cart systems and are beginning to use them to customize their sites to appeal to individual users' preferences. Cookies cannot be used to retrieve other information off your hard drive, or to transmit a virus, and they are in no way a security risk. However, many commercial Web sites subscribe to marketing services that use cookies to track your surfing habits, generating a consumer profile that is potentially available to all the sites that have signed up with the marketing service. If you don't like the idea of this

---

masters, geeks at my service provider, etc.) tell about me—does someone know what pages I access, and when?"

The answer is that yes, your surfing habits can be tracked, and certainly there are marketers eager to capitalize on this information, just as there are print catalogers eager to bombard you with junk mail every time you place a mail order. But you have far more control over how much of your personal data appears online than you might realize (see the "Privacy Tips" sidebar, p. 198, for details). And for up-to-date information on legislation, technology, and your consumer rights, you have valuable online resources such as the Electronic Privacy Information Center (EPIC), The Electronic Frontier Foundation (EFF), and The Center for Democracy and Technology, all of which advocate for individual rights to privacy. As technology grows more sophisticated, it's likely that you'll have considerable control over your personal information and will be able to provide it as selectively as you choose.

Of course, rather than fretting over privacy violations, you do have the

kind of monitoring taking place unbeknownst to you, you can set your browser to either warn you about cookies or refuse to accept them.

Insist on confidentiality. Before you give your e-mail address, street address, or phone number to a company doing business on the Web, check into their confidentiality policy. If you don't receive a guarantee that they won't sell, rent, or trade your information to another business, you may want to go elsewhere.

Think ahead. Choose any passwords carefully, and don't make obvious choices—for example, don't use your mother's maiden name or your daughter's birth date. Keep your passwords written down in a safe place that's not easily accessible to others.

Encrypt. If you're not comfortable with the possibility that the e-mail or files you send online could be intercepted and read by another individual, you might want to encrypt your correspondence. Encryption software—the same type of programs used to secure credit card transac-

tions online—encodes your message, which can then be unscrambled only by the recipient. For information on encryption software, as well as news updates related to governmental efforts to control encryption, check out the Internet Privacy Coalition or the Electronic Privacy Information Center (EPIC).

Fight spam. Spam—the term popularly used for the online equivalent of junk mail sent to individual or group mailing lists—is not exactly an invasion of privacy, but it's definitely a nuisance. Spam costs you money (since it ties up your server and fills up your mailbox) and wastes your time. Not only can't you control whether or not you receive this unsolicited mail, but you frequently can't respond to it, since many spammers use a fake return address. The issue of spam control is being addressed on the federal level, but individual ISPs—some of which filter out spam for their customers—are having more success dealing with this relatively benign irritation. You can research your own ISP's policies and visit an antispamming site for more assistance.

option of adopting the attitude that you have nothing to hide. Granted, we've made a career out of talking about a topic that most folks have been socialized to keep under their hats, so it's easy for us to speak openly about chasing sex links all over the Web. But given how many of your friends, neighbors, and co-workers are doing the same, would it really be so embarrassing to stand up and be counted as someone who seeks sex information and relishes sex entertainment?

Sure, you're justified in not wanting to receive a deluge of spam from "Hot Spicy Babes" just because you filled out a survey or ordered a sex toy. And we understand that you might not want your co-workers identifying your discussion board postings about anal lubricants. Still, we can't help dreaming of the day when sexuality will be so normalized that you would be pleased to have a cookie on your computer indicate that the Good Vibrations site features a red silicone dildo that exactly matches the red jeans you just ordered from J. Crew, or thrilled to have an office mate pull you aside to say that she agreed wholeheartedly with your posted review of the latest Nina Hartley video.

Censorship

The shadow of the Communications Decency Act continues to loom over all issues of free speech and censorship online. Passed in late 1995, the CDA criminalized "indecent" materials on the Web, with the result that a huge range of sites—from those related to breast self-exams to those devoted to Renaissance art—were potentially illegal. In 1997 the Supreme Court ruled that the CDA was so sweepingly vague that it was in clear violation of the First Amendment. But the argument that fueled the CDA— We Must Protect the Nation's Children from Pornography!—is now fueling the latest efforts to restrict access to sexually explicit materials on the Web. And these efforts could result in censorship on an even broader scale than previously imagined.

Filters
One of the best-known tools for restricting children's access to adult sites is filtering software. We gave a brief overview of some of the limitations of filters in chapter 5, "Parenting and Sex Education." These clumsy tools narrow the field of what's available online to a degree that is almost ludicrous—some filters block entire ISPs for the sake of blocking one or two sites, and EPIC has reported that the popular filtering program Net Shepherd leaves users with access to less than 10 percent of the material on

the Web. As a result, legal battles are currently under way around the country to determine whether it's a violation of the First Amendment to mandate filtering software in libraries and schools, since filters inevitably screen out constitutionally protected material.

We respect the fact that parents and educators have a right to limit children's access to X-rated materials. The trouble with filtering software and the rating systems we'll discuss in the following section is that they exceed the limitations placed on minors in the offline world. Surely it's possible to develop restrictions that more closely approximate the rules of the game offline, in which minors simply aren't allowed to buy a *Hustler* magazine or rent a porn video (we may not believe that doing either of these things would be damaging to a child, but we accept the fact that technically it's illegal). Adult pay sites and sites that use adult verification services (an "AVS" provides passwords to thousands of sites for a single fee) already limit access to those old enough to have a credit card. Of course, there will always be ways for kids to get around these restrictions, and currently it's not difficult to find graphic images on free sites and banner ads—if you are looking for them. But we're pretty sure that most of you had the opportunity to scope out a pornographic magazine well before you reached the age of eighteen and that you probably emerged from the experience untraumatized. We believe that kids who do wind up viewing a banner ad for the "Twat Connection" or "Pussy with Pizazz" will be similarly unharmed—especially if they also have access to valuable sex information and educational materials.

Labels and Rating

A proposed solution to the "problem" of sexually explicit material online, one that is gaining in popularity, is based on a labeling technology known as PICS, which stands for Platform for Internet Content Selection. PICS is simply a language that can encode labels into a site, so that different rating organizations can easily search and filter out sites based on a variety of criteria (most filtering software relies in part on PICS). Site owners can use it to rate their sites however they choose, or third-party organizations can use it to rate sites based on their own criteria and values. Proponents of PICS argue that the technology is value-neutral and empowers individuals, since it can be used to support a whole range of rating systems; for example, parents could hypothetically choose between a rating system tailored by the ACLU or one tailored by the Christian Coalition.

If you've visited the sites listed in this book (which we sure hope you have by now), you've probably noticed that many have registered with the major filtering companies and many also carry a RSACi logo. RSAC stands for the Recreational Software Advisory Council, which started out as an organization rating video games and has since expanded its purview to include Web sites (the "i" in RSACi is for Internet). Adult site owners voluntarily rate themselves on a scale of one to four in the categories of sex, nudity, violence, and language and receive a corresponding RSACi label that is encoded in their site. RSACi is an example of the kind of self-rating program that proponents of rating systems argue will make it possible for browsers and search engines equipped with PICS to filter sites more selectively than filtering software does now.

The trouble with self-rating programs is that most sites don't fit into neat categories (level two for violence; level three for nudity). As the folks at the online magazine *mouth organ* note in an article entitled "Why We Don't Rate, and Other Net Effects," "There is no room in RSAC's taxonomy for the site that talks about sex. All the questions on the RSAC site are geared toward the mentality of 'how filthy is your porn?' We don't have any porn at all . . . but then again, we have discussed, at one point or another, all of the most taboo topics on RSAC's lists. So we are in the ludicrous position of being simultaneously one of RSAC's cleanest candidates and one of its filthiest."

The civil liberties organizations that are lining up to oppose rating systems point out that with so few sites rating themselves, any program or browser that blocks unrated sites will block almost the entire Web—from e-zines like *mouth organ* to major news organizations like the *New York Times*. And third-party rating is so labor-intensive that it's entirely possible that a couple of monolithic systems could come to dominate the field, earning a spot as the default rating system for browsers, search engines, online service providers such as AOL, or even governments, which could choose to censor their citizens' access to certain parts of the Web.

We ourselves have an abiding suspicion of labels, which we come by honestly after a decade of selling sex toys, books, and videos. During our tenure at Good Vibrations, we sold a lot of explicit written and visual erotica that didn't get the wide exposure it deserved, and we saw a lot of written and visual material diluted to ensure wider distribution. In this country, the marketplace imposes preemptive self-censorship on sexual materials. Wal-Mart refuses to carry CDs with certain labels, which leads record companies to excise potentially offensive lyrics. Blockbuster Video refuses to stock NC-17 and X-rated tapes, so directors struggle over edits that will earn them an R rating. It hardly seems far-fetched that any Web site striving to satisfy the rating criteria of a behemoth like Netscape or Yahoo! will practice the same type of self-censorship.

RANT: KIDDIE PORN?

To say that we live in a sex-negative society is an understatement. At all levels—individual, cultural, and political—we're socialized to focus on the negative consequences of sex. As vibrator saleswomen, we got used to fielding anxious queries whenever we suggested that enjoying a sex toy might expand a customer's sexual horizons or provide a reliable, abundant source of sexual pleasure: Will I get addicted? Will it replace my partner? Will I have too much pleasure? Similarly, the fact that the Web offers an abundant source of sex-related information and entertainment has been overshadowed from the get-go by anxiety that it must therefore also offer an abundance of the most negative kind of sexual material: child pornography. And the fact that parents' groups and politicians are working to restrict children's access to pornography on the Web is widely interpreted to mean that children are the subjects of pornography on the Web!

Everyone's familiar with the stereotype of the Web as a pervert's paradise, in which child pornographers and pedophiles roam freely, preying on the young and innocent. Yet child pornography is not commercially available in the United States, and any and all distribution is vigorously prosecuted by the Feds: in fact, it's strictly illegal to show any images (photos or drawings) of explicit nudity or sexual acts involving minors, even if the acts are simulated. You might be able to track down images of underage nude models or minors engaged in sexual activity on the Web (probably from overseas sites), but these make up an extremely tiny fraction of the explicit material that's online—which in turn makes up a small fraction of all the material that's online. Unfortunately, unscrupulous adult site owners who rely on misleading banners such as "100 Percent Teen Sex" or "Suite Sex Teen" to generate hits only fuel the stereotype.

As a result of these popular misconceptions, honorable members of the adult industry have become so defensive that adult webmasters go to the somewhat ludicrous lengths of creating and joining organizations such as ASACP, "Adult Sites Against Child Porn." Member sites who sign up for free with this organization can proudly post its logo (and many of the sites reviewed in this book do just that), proclaiming to the world that their site doesn't "contain or condone" child pornography. Maybe you think there's a logical connection between adult materials and kiddie porn, but when was the last time you saw a bakery proudly post a sign announcing that it was against eating disorders or an auto dealership advertise that it was against hit-and-run drivers? If increased access to sexual materials via the Web does nothing else, we hope it will counteract some of the societal biases that make it so hard for us to distinguish between sexual expression and sexual abuse.

Proponents of PICS-based rating systems sing the praises of a brave new Web where you could custom-blend the specifications of your filter so that you would never have to encounter any sites that you might find disturbing. Don't want your kids accessing sites related to porn, drugs, or gambling? Don't want to run across sites devoted to racist, anti-Semitic, or gay-bashing rhetoric? Well, presto!—just screen them out.

Maybe we are a bit old-fashioned, but what ever happened to the concept of free will? Do we really need to program our computers to protect us from ideas, words, or images that we find objectionable? Since when did we become so sensitive that we can't bear to be reminded that these ideas even exist? Sure, the Web is a powerful technology, but the last time we checked, no webmaster was capable of reaching out through the screen and holding a gun to our heads. If we're comfortable turning off the TV or radio when we don't like what's on, surely we can similarly exit sites that offend us. It will be a sad thing indeed if the technology that has offered exposure to a wider realm of ideas and information than any single medium before devolves into a environment that is dictated entirely by personal tastes—and ultimately, perhaps, by the lowest common denominator of taste.

Onward

High-tech and governmental organizations may be duking it out over how best to monitor content, privacy, and control of the Web, but for now it remains a medium that can't really be contained or managed by any regulatory body. To a certain extent, it is still the property and playground of its users: surfers like you. We hope that what you've read in this book has given you a greater sense of the infinite resources available to you on the Web and that it inspires you to be wary of any attempts to limit your access to these resources. We also hope that it's stimulated your erotic imagination.

Many of the women we spoke to while working on this book described how their online experiences enhanced their self-knowledge and increased their acceptance of their own sexual feelings, desires, and fantasies. As this survey respondent expresses eloquently, the kind of self-acceptance you may find online can be powerfully transformative: "When you stop questioning the validity of such a personal part of yourself [as your sexuality], it makes you a lot more willing to think that you've got a clue regarding everything else in your life. Conversely, if you can be made to feel conspicuous and freaky for something as personal as sex, you are a lot less willing to believe your perceptions in other ways."

The Web is what you choose to make of it, and it's only an interactive medium if you decide to interact. Contact other women whose sites you've enjoyed, try your hand at some erotic writing, participate in some online forums . . . and then take everything you learn about your sexual feelings, desires, and fantasies and have fun incorporating that new self-knowledge into your offline life.

We hope you'll come visit us at our Web site. Until then, enjoy!

Reviews

Anonymizer

http://www.anonymizer.com

When you sign up with this site to "cloak" your online travel, the Web sites you visit will not be able to identify your computer or hand you cookies; the downside is that it disables Java and Java Script—which limits your access to certain features such as chat—and it can make surfing slower.

The Center for Democracy and Technology

http://www.cdt.org/privacy

This site's privacy page demonstrates what information can be tracked on your visit to any Web site and explains how it's done.

Cookie Central

http://www.cookiecentral.com

Comprehensive, easy-to-understand and up-to-date information on cookie technology, its uses, and its possible abuses.

Grrltalk

http://www.grrltalk.net/flooding.html

Includes a gateway that allows you to check your own finger information.

The Electronic Privacy Information Center (EPIC)

http://www.epic.org

Offers information about a range of privacy-related issues on the Internet.

The Internet Privacy Coalition

http://www.privacy.org/ipc

Dedicated to promoting privacy and security on the Internet through making encryption tools widely available.

Netizens Against Gratuitous Spamming (NAGS)

http://www.nags.org

Learn technical solutions to the problem of spamming (with tutorials) and read up on the pros and cons of some of the legal solutions currently under consideration. Good links to other antispam sites.

TRUSTe

http://www.truste.com

A nonprofit that uses its privacy assurance program to audit Web site privacy practices.

FREE SPEECH

The Censorship Files

http://www.clairescorner.com/censorship

If you get a bit weary of free-speech polemics, surf over to this excellent, well-balanced links site devoted to the First Amendment and the written word. You'll find sections on banned books and on censorship on the Internet, articles about censorship that reflect an impressive range of attitudes, information on Banned Books Week (an annual event sponsored by libraries and booksellers in the United States), censorship discussion boards, and information on where to buy banned books. The Internet section is not as comprehensive as other link sites in this chapter, but the site as a whole provides a welcome reminder that every free-speech battle being fought in cyberspace was and is still being fought over print books, too.

The Electronic Frontier Foundation (EFF)

http://www.eff.org

Founded in 1990, EFF is a nonprofit civil-liberties organization working to protect privacy, free expression, and democracy online. Their site offers up-to-the-minute news briefs as well as a searchable archive for articles on a range of civil-liberties topics: privacy and encryption, censorship and free speech, legislation and regulation, intellectual property online, and many more. A great resource for information about legislation that will affect your online experience.

Families Against Internet Censorship

http://shell.rmi.net/~fagin/faic

Established by two concerned parents after the CDA's passage, FAIC is dedicated to opposing "those who would use the power of government to regulate Internet content in the name of 'protecting the family'" and to the belief that "parents are the people best suited to decide what their children should and should not see." You'll find a list of member families in almost every one of the fifty states, as well as in other countries—many member families provide personal statements about why they oppose Internet censorship. While the site hasn't been updated since the CDA was overturned, it remains a moving testament to free speech and a valuable read for parents who may be concerned about these issues. It contains links to other anticensorship organizations and filtering software, with the caveat that you "carefully investigate how these programs work and what sites they block to make sure their judgments are ones you agree with."

Feminists for Free Expression (FFE)

http://www.well.com/user/freedom

Don't miss this organization's clearly written, well-constructed series of postings on free speech and feminism (topics include arts censorship, the Internet, sexual harassment, and pornography). You'll also find a roster of the feminist spokeswomen who make up the FFE Speakers Bureau, a veritable who's who of free speech and sex activists, all of whom are available to discuss anticensorship with media, professional and political organizations, colleges, and universities. Alas, our only caveat about this site is that it is infrequently updated and probably won't inspire repeat visits.

Feminists for Free Expression is "a group of diverse feminists working to preserve the individual's right and responsibility to read, listen, view and produce materials of her choice, without the intervention of the state 'for her own good.'" We love this organization because its sex-positive, politically savvy members have been in the trenches since 1992, defending the right to all forms of sexual and artistic expression in their battles against local, state, and national legislation that threatens free speech.

If you've ever felt qualms about whether enjoying pornography is consonant with being a feminist, you owe it to yourself to surf right over to FFE's site and read the text of their beautifully written brochure, "Feminism and Free Speech: Pornography," which responds to the myth that "pornography degrades women," using impeccable reasoning: "Sexism, not sex, degrades women. Though sexism pervades our culture in many forms, we will not eliminate it by banning sex. Sexism and violence stem from long-standing economic, political and emotional factors. It is these that need addressing."

FFE was active in the successful court challenge of the CDA, filing a brief that focused on all the ways in which banning "indecent" materials would deny women access to valuable information, such as breast self-exams, safer-sex techniques, and discussions of rape, domestic violence, and sexual abuse. When we asked Joan Kennedy Taylor, vice-president of the FFE board of directors, whether she thought restrictions on sexual content online had relaxed since that battle, she replied, "No. I was at the Internet Online Summit [held in December 1997], and the impression I got was that the ISPs were so scared of censorship that they were running to self-censor. For instance, Janet Reno announced a policy of 'zero-tolerance' for child pornography and immediately the rumor spread that one ISP had sent a letter to all the others saying that now we must take steps to remove all S/M materials from our customers' sites (S/M being neither child porn nor obscene)."

While FFE is against mandating filtering systems, their position is that individual parents may want to make use of blocking software in the home, and Joan notes that "bad as they are, they are somewhat better than proposed content rating systems and browser design that would skip over unrated sites."

FFE fiercely protects and freely celebrates all forms of sexual expression, and you're not likely to find any other anticensorship or feminist group with so many sex writers, activists, and workers on board. The FFE Speakers Bureau, which sponsors speaking engagements at universities and with the media, includes luminaries such as Candida Royalle, Carol Queen, Pat Califia, Betty Dodson, and Nancy Friday, all of whom are persuasive advocates for the principle that "feminism doesn't stand for censorship."

Has Your Site Been Banned?

http://www.io.com/~vitale/ban

Sidra Vitale, one of the founding members of Web by Women for Women, has put up a rousing polemic against filtering software that includes valuable links to the filtering policies and criteria of organizations such as CyberPatrol, CyberSitter, SurfWatch, and Net Nanny, as well as links to free-speech information and organizations. She has instituted the Banned Sites Web Ring for sites such as hers that don't make it past the filters.

Internet Free Expression Alliance

http://www.ifea.net

The Alliance is an organization of free speech advocates who oppose mandated rating systems of filters, pointing out that "any rating that exists solely to allow specific content to be blocked from view may inhibit the flow of free expression." You'll find regular news updates, links to member organizations, and an excellent collection of resources (articles, position papers, and court summaries) related to legal and technological threats to free speech online.

Peacefire

http://www.peacefire.org

"The youth alliance against Internet censorship," Peacefire is a gold mine of resources related to Internet content legislation, filtering software, and rating systems. These teens know their stuff, they are dedicated to representing the interests of students and minors, and they make a persuasive case for "free speech, equal youth rights and the opportunity for young people to view material online without interference." While Peacefire makes absolutely no bones about its opposition to blocking software (featuring a "blocked site of the day" on the site), consumers of all ideologies can benefit from the site's comparison of the different filtering softwares currently available and how they work. We were particularly impressed by the excellent array of up-to-date news briefs and archives of the same.

Sex Laws

http://www.geocities.com/Capitol Hill/2269

This collection of links to assorted state, federal, and international penal codes related to sex crimes is not annotated, so all you get are the bare facts. You may be shocked to discover how the penalties for serious crimes such as sexual assault vary from place to place, yet how many states still have laws on the books criminalizing oral and anal sex between consenting adults! Lewdness, indecency, sodomy, obscenity, and crimes against nature— you'll find statutes defining all of these, seldom consistently (about nineteen states are covered). Don't miss the excellent links to related sites, for information on everything from parental consent laws on abortion to the history of zoophilia laws.

Web by Women for Women

http://www.io.com/~wwwomen

Subtitled "Fighting Censorship That Affects Women," this grassroots site is guaranteed to make every red-blooded American female proud (and not just because the stars and stripes are waving on the homepage). Who among us is not inspired by the words "We protest all the social and legal pressures that leave women and girls thinking that perfectly normal bodily processes are shameful, evil, pornographic, or topics to only be spoken of in embarrassed whispers and euphemisms to the school nurse."

Compiled by a small group of women outraged by the fact that topics such as breast cancer, abortion, and contraception were temporarily declared "indecent" after the CDA was passed, the site includes articles and essays revealing the time-honored ways in which women's health and sexual well-being are the first casualties of any attempts to "protect" us from "indecency." The site is also home to the range of essays on sexuality described on p. 96

Glossary

Bandwidth. The amount of data that can be transmitted through any online channel, measured in bits per second.

Banner ads. Advertisements that appear in banner form across your screen; you can click on the banner to go to the site being advertised.

BDSM. Acronym for a variety of sexual practices or fantasies involving power exchange: B/D refers to bondage and discipline, D/S to dominance and submission, and S/M to sadomasochism.

Bit. Short for binary digit, the smallest unit of computer data.

Bookmark. A browser tool that allows you to save any Web address in a file for future reference.

Browser. Navigation software that provides the graphical interface between your computer and the Web.

Chat. Online text-based communication that takes place instantaneously, in real time.

Click-through. A marketing gimmick designed to transport you from the site you chose to visit to another that will kick back a small payment to the original site. Click-throughs can take the form of a visible banner ad or a hidden link within a site.

Conference. An online discussion forum in which participants read and post messages on a topic of shared interest. Conferences are time-delayed, not instantaneous, forms of communication.

Cookie. A piece of data about your visit to a Web site that the site stores on your computer's hard drive to access upon your return. You'll often hear people refer to being "handed a cookie" by a site.

CU–SeeMe. A software used for video conferencing (trademarked by White Pine).

Directory. An online research tool in which site listings are categorized by subject matter; many search engines also maintain directories.

Domain name. The part of a Web address that is the identifying name chosen and registered by the individual, company, or organization that created the site.

D/S. Sexual practices or fantasies involving dominant and submissive role-playing.

FAQ. Frequently Asked Questions; many sites offer a FAQ section as an introduction to basic content.

Femdom or femdomme. Short for female dominant. One of several abbreviations to identify BDSM role-playing preferences. You'll also see the terms maledom, femsub, and malesub.

Flame. To respond to someone's posted comments with a posting that attacks, insults, or provokes: it's a flame because it generates a lot of heat. The word can be used as a noun or a verb.

FTP or File Transfer Protocol. A text-based protocol for sending and retrieving files (that can contain either text or images) between computers via the Internet.

Gopher. A text-only, menu-driven protocol that allows you to search for and retrieve information from the Internet (you are "burrowing" through a web of gopher sites).

Handle. A term adopted from CB radio, a handle is an online pseudonym.

Homepage. The entry page or table of contents page for any Web site, the homepage often contains a general introduction to the site.

HTML. The acronym for Hypertext Markup Language, the language code used to create Web sites.

Hyperlink (or link). An embedded element in a hypertext file that allows you to move around within a Web site or from one site to another with a point and click.

Hypertext. A cross-referenced file containing links that allow you to move from file to file in a nonlinear fashion.

ICQ. Software that provides Web-based instant messaging, friend recognition, and real-time chat.

IRC or Internet Relay Chat. Worldwide text-based, real-time chat taking place on specific Internet channels. Not accessible through the Web without specific software and access to an ISP that is part of an IRC network.

ISP or Internet Service Provider. A company with a centralized computer system that offers users access to the Internet for a fee.

Java. The programming language used to create many of the interactive features of Web sites.

Listserv. An e-mail mailing list in which all subscribers receive postings related to a topic of common interest; subscription to a listserv is usually free.

Live streaming video (or live feed). Transmission of real-time video images onto your computer screen. In adult streaming video you pay by the minute to view sexual performances, and you can direct and interact with the performer(s) by typing commands and comments back and forth.

Lurk. To hang out in a chat room or read the postings in a conference without participating in the discussion.

MUDs. Text-based, interactive, multiplayer adventure games involving real-time chat. Not accessible through the Web without specific client software and access to a host server.

Netiquette. Online courtesy (from "net" plus "etiquette").

Netizen. Anyone who spends time online (from "net" plus "citizen").

Offline. Where you are when you're not online! Also known as real life, or RL.

Polyamory. Multipartner relationships; often referred to as responsible nonmonogamy.

Protocol. The language or format used to transmit files over the Internet.

Search engine. An online research tool that sifts through the Web to retrieve data based on specific key words or phrases.

Slash. A genre of erotic fan fiction revolving around popular TV characters (from shows such as *Star Trek* or *The X-Files*) that often has a homoerotic theme.

S/M. Sexual practices or fantasies involving power exchange. The abbreviation S/M originally derived from the term *sadomasochism*, but you'll also hear it referred to as "sexual magic." The slash between the S and the M signifies the fluidity between and interdependence of the two poles of role-playing.

Spam. The flooding of any medium—whether private e-mail, conferences, IRC, or Usenet newsgroups—with inappropriate chatter, solicitations, or information. Often used in reference to electronic junk mail or excessive multiple postings to newsgroups.

Thread. A continuous chain of postings on a single topic in a conference or newsgroup.

Thumbnail. Images—usually photos—that load in miniature; you can click on the thumbnail of your choice to see the image at a larger size.

Transgendered. An umbrella term for individuals whose identity and experience don't conform to traditional gender roles, including transsexuals, cross-dressers, and intersexed people.

URL. The address for a Web site. URL stands for Uniform Resource Locator.

Usenet newsgroups. Internet conferences in which participants read and post messages on a topic of shared interest. Newsgroups predate the Web.

Video conferencing. Exchanging video images transmitted over the Internet, so that users can chat or perform on each other's computer screens in real time.

Web ring. An informal linking of sites that are related in theme or philosophy.

Zine. A low-budget, low-gloss publication that often serves as a mouthpiece for one or two opinionated editors.

Index

Adam & Eve, 126, 139
Adam and Gillian's Sensual Whips and Toys, 147
addresses, Web, 7–8
advice columns, 83, 102–7
Airs, Kim, 132, 135
All About Sex, 120–21
Alman, Isadora, 105, 158, 178–79, 180–81
Altmann, Madeleine, 54, 57–62, 63
alt.sex column, 102, 105–6
amateur sex sites, 55–57, 75–76
American Sex Machines, 85–86
America Online (AOL), 4, 106
anal sex, 105–6
Angela Preston (site name: X-stories), 32
Anne and Cathy's Home Page, 65
Anne Rose's Ultimate Birth Control Links, 189–90
Anne's Erotic Story Archives, 14–15, 32
anonymity, 14–15, 82–83, 198–200, 205
Anonymizer, 205
Anything That Moves, 40
aphrodisiacs, 91
Ars Magna Erotica, 23, 33
Art and Love on the Net, 175
art and photography, 23–24, 33–34
arts and entertainment, 11–50
ASACP, 203
Ashe, Danni, 54, 57–62, 69–70
Asia Carerra's XXX Buttkicking Homepage, 71, 73–74
Ask Delilah, 102–3
Ask Dr. Myrtle, 106, 138

Ask Me Anything, 103
Ask the Couch!, 103, 106
Authoritative Matchmaker, 185
Auto Erotic House of Art, 33–34
Axfords Corset Catalogue, 148

Babes4U, 57–62, 70
bandwidth, 3, 173
banner ads, 62
Barbach, Lonnie, 12
Barnard, Ellen, 132
BDSM, 81, 147–51
Belton, Todd, 21
Benedicks, Adrienne, 14–15, 16, 17, 18
Bernadette Taylor: The Diary of a Virtual Girlfriend, 76
Best American Erotica, 126
Better Business Bureau, 64, 77, 127, 129
Bianca's Smut Shack, 179–80
birth control, 82, 98, 112, 189–90
Bisexual Internet Resources, 190
bisexuals, 81, 82, 118, 171, 190
Blank, Joani, 131
Block, Dr. Susan, 23, 141
Blowfish: Good Products for Great Sex, 140
Body: Safe Sex and Prevention, 98
bookmark, 7
books and videos, 143–47
Brame, Gloria Glickstein, 66, 160; Castle in the Sky, 66
Brat Attack, 21, 41
Bright, Susie, 52, 66–67, 160